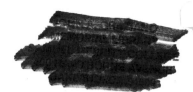

User Education
in Health Sciences Libraries
A Reader

11/8/95

HAWORTH Medical Information Sources
M. Sandra Wood, MLS, MBA
Senior Editor

New, Recent, and Forthcoming Titles:

How to Find Information About AIDS, 2nd Edition
edited by Jeffrey T. Huber

*CD-ROM Implementation and Networking in Health Sciences
Libraries* edited by M. Sandra Wood

User Education in Health Sciences Libraries: A Reader
by M. Sandra Wood

User Education in Health Sciences Libraries
A Reader

M. Sandra Wood, MLS, MBA
Editor

The Haworth Press
New York • London

The Haworth Press, Inc., 10 Alice Street, Binghamton, NY 13904-1580

Library of Congress Cataloging-in-Publication Data

User education in health sciences libraries : a reader / M. Sandra Wood, editor.
    p.   cm.
   Includes bibliographical references and index.
   ISBN 1-56024-995-1 (pbk : alk paper)
   1. Medical libraries–United States. 2. Library orientation–United States. I. Wood, M. Sandra.
Z675.M4U83   1995
026.61–dc20   95-30629
                                                       CIP

CONTENTS

PART IV. INFORMATION MANAGEMENT EDUCATION
AND COMPUTER LITERACY PROGRAMS

ABOUT THE EDITOR

M. Sandra Wood, MLS, MBA, is Librarian, Reference and Database Services, at The Milton S. Hershey Medical Center of The Pennsylvania State University at Hershey. She holds the academic rank of Librarian and has over 24 years of experience as a medical reference librarian, including general reference services, management of reference services, database searching, and user instruction. As an experienced medical reference librarian, as well as online search analyst, Ms. Wood has published widely in the field of medical reference and is Editor of the journal *Medical Reference Services Quarterly*. She is active in the Medical Library Association and Special Libraries Association, most recently serving on MLA's Board of Directors as Treasurer.

CONTRIBUTORS

Francesca Allegri, MS, Consultant, Charlotte, NC.

Carol M. Antoniewicz, MLS, Reference Librarian, Todd Wehr Library, Medical College of Wisconsin Libraries.

Glynis Vandoorne Asu, AMLS, Interlibrary Loan Librarian, Medical College of Wisconsin Libraries.

helen-ann brown, MLS, MS, Information Services Team, Samuel J. Wood Library/C. V. Starr Biomedical Information Center, Cornell University Medical College.

Joyce J. Bryant, Library Assistant/Interlibrary Loan Specialist, Scott Memorial Library, Thomas Jefferson University.

Melinda Buckwalter, BA, Microcomputer Room Staff, Samuel J. Wood Library/C. V. Starr Biomedical Information Center, Cornell University Medical College.

Judy F. Burnham, MLS, Assistant Librarian and UMC Site Coordinator, Biomedical Library, University of South Alabama, Mobile.

Mitchell Aaron Cahan, MLS, formerly Personal Information Management Specialist, William H. Welch Medical Library, Johns Hopkins University School of Medicine. He is now a medical student at Johns Hopkins.

Nancy Calabretta, MEd, Sharp Health Science Library, Cooper Hospital, University Medical Center, Camden, NJ.

Dudee Chiang, MS, CAS, Thomas and Dorothy Leavey Library, University of Southern California.

Stephen Clancy, MLS, Reference Librarian, Science Library, University of California, Irvine.

Barbara Collins, MSLS, Microcomputer Librarian, Paul Himmelfarb Health Sciences Library, George Washington University Medical Center, Washington, DC.

Margaret Devlin, MLS, Director, Rohrbach Library, Kutztown University, Pennsylvania.

Sandra C. Dow, AMLS, formerly Head Librarian, Public Health Library, University of Michigan.

Jonquil D. Feldman, MLS, formerly Consultation Services Coordinator, The Claude Moore Health Sciences Library, University of Virginia.

Jacqueline Glick, MLS, Head of User Services, Medical College of Wisconsin Libraries.

Beverly A. Gresehover, MLS, Consultant, Information Crossroads, Columbia, MD.

David N. King, PhD, Special Assistant for Information Education, Library and Center for Knowledge Management, University of California, San Francisco.

Julia K. Kochi, MILS, Library Associate, National Library of Medicine, Washington, DC.

Barbara Laynor, MSLS, Scott Memorial Library, Thomas Jefferson University.

Beth Layton, MLS, MBA, Head of Information Services, William H. Welch Medical Library, Johns Hopkins University.

Anne Linton, MS, Associate Director of Information, Instructional and Media Services, Paul Himmelfarb Health Sciences Library, George Washington University Medical Center, Washington, DC.

Barbara Lucas, MLS, Reference Librarian, Science Library, University of California, Irvine.

Joanne G. Marshall, PhD, Associate Professor, Faculty of Information Studies, University of Toronto.

Jonathan Merril, MD, Co-founder & Chief Technology Officer, High Techsplanations Inc., Rockville, MD.

Elizabeth Mikita, MLS, Bibliographic Management and Automation Librarian, the Scott Memorial Library, Thomas Jefferson University.

Rochelle L. Minchow, MLS, Medical Education Curriculum Coordinator, Science Library, University of California, Irvine.

Craig Mulder, MILS, Health Sciences Librarian, Michigan State University Libraries.

Janet L. Nelson, MLS, Information Specialist and Bibliographic Instruction Coordinator, Norris Medical Library, University of Southern California.

Karyn Pomerantz, MLS, User Education Librarian, Paul Himmelfarb Health Sciences Library, George Washington University Medical Center, Washington, DC.

Kathryn Pudlock, MLS, formerly Reference Librarian, the Biomedical Library of the University of California, Irvine.

Peggy W. Richwine, MS, MLS, Reference Librarian, Ruth Lilly Medical Library, Indiana University.

Diane G. Schwartz, MLS, Associate Director for Medical Education/Research Associate Professor of Medicine, Primary Care Resource Center, State University of New York at Buffalo.

Phyllis C. Self, PhD, Director, Tompkins-McCaw Library, Medical College of Virginia, Virginia Commonwealth University.

James Shedlock, AMLS, Director, Galter Health Sciences Library, Northwestern University, Chicago.

Barbara Lowther Shipman, AMLS, Head, Electronics Information Systems, Alfred Taubman Medical Library, University of Michigan.

Dan Sienkiewicz, BFA, Microcomputer Specialist, Samuel J. Wood Library/C. V. Starr Biomedical Information Center, Cornell University Medical College.

Bernie Todd Smith, MSLS, Director, Werner Health Sciences Library, Rochester General Hospital.

Julia Sollenberger, MLS, Assistant Director, Edward G. Miner Library, School of Medicine and Dentistry, University of Rochester, NY.

Kathleen Strube, MLS, Manager of Library Services, Aurora Medical Library Services, Aurora Health Care, St. Luke's Medical Center, Wisconsin.

JoAnn H. Switzer, MLS, Acting Director, Center for Higher Education and Workforce Development, Indianapolis.

Edward W. Tawyea, MLS, University Librarian and Director, Scott Memorial Library, Thomas Jefferson University.

Virginia Tiefel, AMLS, Director of Library User Education, Ohio State University Libraries.

Nicholas G. Tomaiuolo, Coordinator of Education Programs, Lyman Maynard Stowe Library, University of Connecticut Health Center.

Elizabeth Warner, MSLS, AHIP, Education Services Librarian, Scott Memorial Library, Thomas Jefferson University.

Sally Winthrop, Online Services Coordinator, Paul Himmelfarb Health Sciences Library, George Washington University Medical Center, Washington, DC.

Elizabeth H. Wood, MBA, MSLS, Head, Research & Reference Services and Customer Support, Oregon Health Sciences University Libraries, Portland, OR.

Martha Jane K. Zachert, DLS, Consultant, Tallahassee, FL.

Preface

Educating health professionals and students to be effective, efficient users of biomedical and health sciences information probably began in earnest in the 1960s. When the MEDLARS databases were introduced in the 1970s, health professionals suddenly had a resource to use and contend with that they could never have really fathomed in an earlier time period.

By the early 1980s, library staff had access to personal computers and software which turned those computers into magical tools that opened up a host of potentially new activities and roles for librarians. For the first time, computers were available to perform a variety of functions other than circulation control and collection management. As the potential for the use of those computers became evident, public services librarians in health sciences libraries jumped on the bandwagon of what was known in general academic libraries as the "bibliographic instruction movement."

Bibliographic instruction had become an important professional activity in many academic health sciences and larger hospital libraries by the first half of the 1980s. The movement was not entirely driven by the availability of new technologies; rather, much of the impetus came from public services librarians, who like myself, found themselves answering the same questions over and over again when working at the reference desk. The obvious solution was to find what had brought so many people into the library. In academic health sciences libraries, a class assignment was the most common explanation, and the solution was to identify the instructor and ask her for time to talk to her class about search strategy techniques. That was how many "b.i." careers began.

As computers became more prevalent in health sciences libraries, and as software for those computers became more sophisticated, librarians quickly developed the ability to exploit the technology to its fullest extent. At the same time, developments were taking place over which librarians had no control. In the 1980s, under pressure from the U.S. Congress, the National Library of Medicine provided commercial firms with access to the MEDLARS tapes. As a result, software companies began producing new versions of the MED-LINE database. Some products were developed specifically for search intermediaries, while others offered specialized interfaces to make it possible for end users to perform their own searches. As a result of these developments, some librarians were challenged, and some were threatened. Perhaps it was easier to be threatened and simply to continue to fulfill the same roles librarians had always filled. Conversely, it was an incredible opportunity to undertake the challenge of developing programs to teach health sciences students, faculty, and staff to learn how to conduct their own bibliographic database searches. The result of taking on this challenge was to ensure that librarians continued to be recognized as the database search experts.

Following the process of developing programs to teach end users how to conduct searches, came the need to teach the use of software to help manage the enormous volume of information that users were accumulating. As additional electronic information resources became available, librarians found the demand to learn how to use these programs and services outpaced their ability to respond. Nevertheless, they did respond. New divisions of reference departments sprang up. They were called information management or education divisions. In some libraries new departments with similar names were created. They varied in size, but however they were organized, they reflected the growing importance of the time and effort being devoted to intructional activites in health sciences libraries.

Another factor which greatly influenced the level of effort health sciences librarians were devoting to educational activities was the publication of the 1984 report *Physicians for the twenty-first century. Report of the Panel on the General Education of the Physician and College Preparation for Medicine.* The report stipulated that medical students learn the skills needed to effectively access and manage biomedical information.

The chapters included in this volume provide an excellent overview of the accomplishments that have taken place in instructional services in health sciences libraries. Many provide insight into the theoretical underpinnings of programs, while others give practical advice for development and implementation. In addition the chapters provide the groundwork for understanding the importance of the librarian's role as instructor, both now and in the future. As librarians assume roles that move them outside the traditional library setting, the ideas shared here will give them the foundation needed to move forward, assume new professional challenges, and succeed in the rapidly changing health information environment.

The chapters span the years 1987-1994, which represent the period of greatest activity in the field, and cover significant diversity in subject matter. This volume will be invaluable to practicing librarians, graduate students seeking to become health sciences librarians, and library administrators seeking to ensure that the programs they are supporting are the best quality.

Diane G. Schwartz

Introduction

M. Sandra Wood

Over the past decade, libraries have been impacted by changing technologies, resulting in new and different roles for librarians. The role of the reference librarian, in particular, has been radically altered due to the rise of end-user searching, the development of information management software, and the creation of the information superhighway. Reference librarians are finding that their role has moved from search intermediary to consultant and educator. It has taken most of the 1980s for this shift to occur. The 1990s will see even more and faster change in the ways that information is accessed, and librarians must be prepared for further change.

In the long run, librarians have always been educators. From the basics of library tours and orientations to instructing about a print index, librarians have taught in one-on-one situations or offered group instruction, as appropriate. On a day-to-day basis, instruction is a routine part of reference services. However, the role of educator is becoming more prominent in the highly technology-oriented environment of the 1990s. The increased need for librarians to educate users means that there is a need for library and information science students and practicing librarians to receive more formal education in teaching theory and methodologies. "Training the trainer" courses have been offered by database producers such as the National Library of Medicine, with the intention of training librarians how to teach their specific product; however, this content-specific training must be supplemented with educational theory and principles. Graduate programs in library and information science usually have geared teaching-related courses specifically to students intending to be school librarians. All graduate students in the field should be taught basic instructional principles in order to fulfill their role as educators, whether they intend to work in an academic, public, school, or special library. Additionally, practicing librarians should be encouraged and offered opportunities to take continuing education courses about instructional methodologies. *Platform for Change: The Educational Policy Statement of the Medical Library Association* (Chicago: MLA, 1989) calls for librarians to possess knowledge and skills in seven broad areas, one of which is Instructional Support Systems. This knowledge area includes learning theory, curriculum development, instructional design, educational needs assessment, learning style appraisal, instructional methodologies, and evaluation of learning objectives.

Given the changing role of reference librarians, this *Reader* is intended to provide ready access to a wide range of articles published about librarians educating users to utilize information resources. The chapters were selected from articles published in *Medical Reference Services Quarterly* from 1987 through 1994. Because of the volume of literature in *MRSQ* related to user education, it was necessary to be highly selective in the articles chosen for this volume. Criteria used for selection were applicability to more than one institution or across all fields of librarianship; currency of information (e.g., product discussed is still available); and uniqueness of the contribution to the literature. The selections include chapters about planning educational programs, educating end-user searchers, teaching about new technology, and utilization of technology for teaching purposes. While the examples are based on experiences in health sciences libraries, the concepts and principles are certainly applicable to other types of libraries.

The volume is divided into five sections, each selectively covering different aspects of user education. Arguably, several of the chapters might have been placed in more than one section. The first section, "Program Planning and Implementation," is concerned with planning for both new and existing programs, and with the implementation of user education programs. These chapters discuss everything from how the programs might fit within the organizational structure to what skills are needed to teach library users. Examples are given of some new and unique programs.

The second section, "Teaching End-User Searching" is concerned with one major area of user education–teaching end users how to search databases. MEDLINE is the featured database, but several chapters discuss searching principles in general, and one concentrates on the changing role of reference librarians as related to database searching. In the third section, "Research in User Education," the first chapter argues the need for research in user education, while the remaining three present research which has been done primarily in the area of database searching.

The fourth section, "Information Management Education and Computer Literacy Programs," moves to another key area in the changing role of user education–information management education (IME). Instruction in computer literacy is closely tied to IME because of the computer skills necessary to utilize IME software. The chapters in this section discuss both IME programs and courses aimed simply at computer literacy. Throughout, the librarian is undertaking new roles as both a consultant and an educator.

In the final section, "Computer-Assisted Instruction and Audio-visual Aids," librarians are utilizing multimedia technologies to facilitate user education. The three chapters present examples of new and different products which have been developed as teaching aids, each using different formats–videotape, computer-assisted instruction, and hypertext.

This volume will have served its purpose if it creates an interest in user education in libraries or generates an idea for a new or expanded user education program. Library and information science students and practitioners can learn from the educational programs that have developed over the last decade, as represented in this volume, to build and expand their role as consultant and educator.

PART I

PROGRAM PLANNING
AND IMPLEMENTATION

Chapter 1

Creating Educational Programs in Libraries: Introduction and Part 1– Training and Education

David N. King

To even mention that information services in health sciences libraries are in transition has become cliché. Our practices of a decade ago seem curiously out-of-date today, and we are confronted with the reality of change on a daily basis. Many of the changes that are occurring reflect necessary responses to the evolving technological environment within which health sciences information is created, stored, disseminated, and used. Perhaps less apparent in this period dominated by electronically facilitated information services are changes that reflect a better understanding of our clientele and a broader conception of our roles as librarians. These changes are prompted, not only by newer technological capabilities, but also by qualitative progress in the subspecialties of information services. Such progress is most easily seen in the development of specialized clinical information services. It is less recognized, if equally remarkable, in the development of innovative instructional programs that have become a requisite part of quality information services in recent years.

Much of the groundwork for the newer instructional programs occurred in the 1970s as librarians began to question the value and

This chapter was first published in *Medical Reference Services Quarterly*, Vol. 6(3), Fall 1987.

motivations of library skills instruction, and to develop programs that were less tool-specific and more educational in nature. Bibliographic instruction, in its most creative manifestations, discarded instruction in such esoteric library details as catalog card filing orders and deciphering index citations, and focused instead on search strategies, structure of the literature, and problem-solving techniques. Bibliographic instruction at its best probably represents the beginnings of educational programming in libraries.

Bibliographic instruction has never become the "movement" in health sciences libraries that it is in general academic libraries. The clientele served by health sciences libraries are typically more advanced academically, have a better grasp of the primary literature, and have different information-seeking styles and needs than college freshmen. Moreover, the librarians in health sciences libraries often hold a different relationship with their clientele and their institution than do their colleagues in general academic libraries. For these reasons, and perhaps also because health sciences libraries have always tipped the balance between providing answers and teaching users to find their own answers in favor of the former, their instructional programs remain primarily skills-training in orientation.

The changes that have taken place in the instructional programs of health sciences libraries in the last few years are more in content than in pedagogy. Instruction in personal files management, online searching for end users, and microcomputer use, among other topics of practical interest to health professionals, have supplemented (sometimes replaced) instruction in the use of library tools. The evolving roles of information services in health sciences libraries, the professional growth of subspecialists concerned with the development of instructional programs, and some hard thinking about user needs and instructional intent, have contributed to these changes and the success with which they have been implemented in many libraries.

Yet, there is still an underlying element of unrealized potential in even the most ambitious and successful programs. The goals of information management education (IME) programs no longer express as their primary intent teaching users about library tools, but rather teaching health professionals effective information-seeking and information-management techniques within the context of their own needs and purposes. IME aspires to transcend the library skills instruction tradition of the past by creating educational programs for their clientele built upon the information management expertise of librarians. The appellation itself, information management *education*, expresses an aspiration to create programs that are more than skills training.

At the current stage of development of IME and other innovative instructional programming in health sciences libraries, it is important to consider some basic concerns about the nature of educational programs and what is required to create successful ones. First, what is it that distinguishes education from training? It is only by answering this question that judgments can be made about the quality of instructional achievements. Second, is education a reasonable and realizable goal for instruction programs in health sciences libraries? Perhaps skills training programs are more appropriate to the needs and interests of health professionals and students in the health sciences, or perhaps there are insurmountable obstacles to creating educational programs in health sciences libraries. And third, what are the costs of educational programs, monetarily, professionally, and administratively? It is only by knowing the costs and comparing them to the benefits that might be derived from educational programs that decisions can be made about the value of the investment.

There are almost as many ways of addressing these concerns as there are libraries and instruction librarians, and each library committed to quality information services will eventually resolve them in its own way. But it is important that they be given due consideration, lest decisions occur by default and opportunities to improve instructional programming in health sciences libraries escape.

In this chapter, some of the characteristics of instructional programs are considered, particularly those that distinguish educational programs from training. In the following two chapters, the feasibility of developing educational programs in health sciences libraries, and the costs of such programs will be addressed. Since instructional practices vary depending upon local circumstances, it is difficult to generalize about them, and impossible to describe the many programs that are offered. Even so, it is useful to employ an example in discussing the issues. Since many libraries currently provide, or plan to offer, instruction in MEDLINE searching for their clientele, either as one component in a course or as a stand-alone workshop, and since most health sciences librarians have received some form of instruction in online searching, this example will be used throughout the discussion.

PART 1: TRAINING AND EDUCATION

Before launching into the distinction between education and training, it is worthwhile to consider how information-seeking and use behaviors and abilities commonly develop. The process by which individuals are socialized into the information networks and communication patterns of their disciplines is not well understood. Research suggests that students tend to model their approaches to research, the literature, and even library use, after faculty and peers whom they would emulate.[1] Librarians seem to play a relatively minor role in the development of information-seeking and information-management behaviors for most students, and consequently for most health professionals. Libraries, the secondary tools which are the principal means of access to the literature in libraries, and the services of librarians, have traditionally been subordinated to less formal approaches to the literature (colleagues) and to the self-indexing nature of the primary literature itself.[2] Even in learning to use libraries, peers and personal experience are usually more influential than librarians for most clientele.

However prevalent this pattern may have been in the past, three trends seem to be inducing change. First, the growth of the literature is disrupting informal approaches to the literature, the ability to remain abreast of relevant literature, and the traditional processes of information control used by health professionals. Second, new technological developments enable individuals to exert more control over their personal information-seeking and information-management systems, and in the process the less formal approaches used in the past are supplanted by approaches that overlap with, or share characteristics with, the more formal approaches employed by libraries. And third, libraries have expanded their efforts to share their professional expertise by seeking the common ground between library practices and knowledge on the one hand, and client needs and behavior on the other. In some cases, librarians either participate in formal instructional programs offered by teaching departments or contribute to planning those programs. It is becoming more common than in the past to see libraries as a direct source of instruction, however.

It is hard to tell how pervasive a force librarians will become in the information-seeking and information-management socialization process for health professionals. If traditional patterns hold true, colleagues, teachers, and published literature which can be consulted personally will continue to serve as major methods for learning. But the recent success of instructional programs for health professionals and students suggest that librarians may play a more prominent role in the learning process. This can be seen in the ways in which people learn to search MEDLINE. Although less formal opportunities for learning to search are available, such as colleagues and literature intended for end users, the number of workshops and courses have not only proliferated, but have also been surprisingly well attended. Formal instruction in academic curricula is becoming more common as well. Unfortunately, most of the instructional programs are predominately training sessions, with little educational content.

In the broadest sense of the term, education includes any activity or other experience which creates the opportunity to learn. A publication, conversation, classroom activity, life experience, or even a period of solitude for reflection could be considered educational. As the term is used here, education refers to a process of developing knowledge and skills which involves systematic consideration of methods and outcomes within a context of principles and theory. Training, in distinction, is used here to refer to a process of developing proficiency in practice or application of knowledge and skills within prescribed circumstances or standards of quality. (There is little consensus concerning the use of these terms, and usage here may not conform to standard definitions.) It should be apparent that training and education are not entirely exclusive; training may include educational elements, and education very often includes training. In instructional practice, the distinction is often more in degree than in kind. Nonetheless, the differences are real, and it is usually

possible to describe a particular instructional effort as primarily
training or as being educational.

The distinction between education and training can be seen in
instruction for online searching of bibliographic databases. Pedagogical differences abound, depending upon local circumstances,
expectations of learners and instructors, motivation and needs of
recipients and providers of instruction, and the goals of the instructional effort. Instruction for end users most frequently emphasizes
the mechanics and procedures of online interaction, use of Boolean
operators, steps in doing a search, and system and database features.
Such instruction often approaches searching as a set of discrete
procedures, commands, and formulae into which the user can insert
terms and in response to which the system will select appropriate
bibliographic citations. Good training for end users also includes
some attention to principles and concepts, but the instruction is
heavily weighted in favor of presenting to learners the rudiments of
basic searching technique. The type of instruction ordinarily provided end users has been described as "operational training."[3]

More extensive is the sort of training typically offered to library
school students and practicing librarians, which is sometimes referred to as "educational training."[3] Such instruction may vary in
intensity and comprehensiveness, depending upon the amount of
time allotted and the prior knowledge of recipients, but the goals
usually reflect higher performance expectations than those posited
for end users. In addition to a more thorough grasp of system and
database features, esoteric commands, and more advanced procedures, educational training often devotes more attention to the use
of terminology and search "tactics."[4] Although the more intensive
training provided by library schools, vendors, and other agencies of
advanced instruction may include greater attention to educational
content than the instruction offered end users, it often does not.
Educational training, except in rare cases, is a misnomer.

Good training and good educational programs share certain important characteristics, certainly. Both are founded upon organized,
systematic consideration of content. Both enable the learner to approach the material according to optimal learning style and at a pace
that optimizes the opportunity to learn. Both present new material
that builds upon the prior knowledge and skills of the learner. But

there are significant differences between training and education as well, both in pedagogy and in purpose. Whereas training aims at developing proficiency in the application of skills, such as the ability to conduct searches at a specific level of excellence, education aims at developing a higher level of knowledge and skills, a level which encompasses the principles upon which practice is based and at which informed enquiry is possible. Whereas in training, the application of skills is the goal, in education the application of skills is but a means to higher ends.

Science students are instructed in the use of laboratory equipment and techniques, not simply to develop proficiency in the instruments of science, but as a means of educating them in the ways of systematic enquiry into the nature of physical phenomena and processes. Philosophy students are instructed in symbolic logic as a tool that can be used for analytical reasoning. Social scientists learn to apply the principles of good questionnaire design, experimental method, and statistics as instruments for controlled enquiry into the human condition. Medical education lays a foundation of biological sciences, not so much because such knowledge is necessary in order to set a broken bone or prescribe an antihistamine, but because the practice of medicine is a conceptual process which requires knowledge of human health and disease processes as a basis for clinical problem solving. The techniques of treatment, even highly sophisticated ones like surgery, are the result of training. Medical education enables the physician to know when a particular treatment is needed, why it is a better choice than another treatment, and how it affects the health and disease process.

The goal of any educational program is to develop problem-solving abilities, not simply to train in particular skills. Information management education, if it is to be an educational rather than a training program, will necessarily transcend skills proficiency as its goal. Where training in online searching emphasizes procedures, education emphasizes process. The formulae and steps of searching are placed in a context of heuristic strategy and tactics. Boolean operators and statement construction become instances of set theory and logic. Selection of terminology defines a scope of knowledge and enquiry. Searching becomes a conceptual process, a problem-solving process, rather than an exercise in operations.

The goal of an IME program, or any component of instruction, if it is to become an educational endeavor, must transcend the goal of training for proficiency in the use of tools and techniques. The goal of information management education, then, is to enable health professionals to master the problem-solving processes and use of particular tools and techniques, such as online searching, for understanding and managing the information process. The feasibility of information management education provided by health sciences libraries, will be considered in Chapter 2.

NOTES

1. Dunn, Kathleen. "Psychological Needs and Source Linkages in Undergraduate Information-Seeking Behavior." In: *Proceedings of the 4th National Conference of the Association of College and Research Libraries.* Edited by Danuta A. Nitecki. Chicago: ACRL, 1986, pp. 172-178.

2. Stoan, Stephen K. "Research and Library Skills: An Analysis and Interpretation." *College and Research Libraries* 45(March 1984):99-109.

3. Wanger, Judith. "Education and Training for Online Systems." *Annual Review of Information Science and Technology* 14(1979):220.

4. Bates, Marcia J. "Information Search Tactics." *Journal of the American Society for Information Science* 30(July 1979):205-214.

Chapter 2

Creating Educational Programs in Libraries: Part 2–Feasibility

David N. King

INTRODUCTION

In the previous chapter, the distinction between training and education was introduced. Training was referred to as instruction aimed at "developing proficiency in practice or application of knowledge and skills within prescribed circumstances or standards of quality." It was suggested that most instruction in health sciences libraries today is of this type. Teaching end users to search served as an example. Such instruction typically presents searching as sets of procedures, commands, system features, and terminological choices, with the intent of providing learners with a rudimentary understanding of search technique. It was also suggested that the sort of instruction received by library school students and librarians, although more intensive and advanced, is training as well. Most other instructional endeavors in health sciences libraries share the characteristics of training; for example, instruction in organizing personal reprint files and use of secondary print tools for information seeking typically focus on basic skills and proficiencies.

In contrast, it was suggested that educational programs endeavor to lay a foundation of principles and theory to guide problem solv-

This chapter was first published in *Medical Reference Services Quarterly*, Vol. 6(4), Winter 1987.

ing and informed enquiry. In educational programs, tools and proficiency in their use become means to higher ends. Searching, for example, becomes a conceptual process rather than an exercise in applying formulae, commands, terms, and procedures. Educational programs in libraries should aim at mastery of problem-solving processes and the use of tools and techniques for managing the information process.

Good training and good educational programs share elements in common. The principles of good instructional design, organization of content, teaching techniques, and so on, apply to both. Moreover, good training often requires educational elements, and good education almost always includes training. In training end users to search, at least a little attention is given to conceptualizing the information need and developing a search strategy. An educational program which includes the use of online systems would be deficient were training not incorporated.

In this chapter, some of the fundamental problems and questions surrounding educational programming in libraries are considered. What would be needed for instruction provided by libraries to transcend training and become educational? What obstacles stand in the way? Is educational programming a reasonable and worthwhile goal for libraries? Is information management *education* really feasible?

FEASIBILITY

In an early evaluation of searching on the MEDLINE system by health professionals, Lancaster identified several areas which seemed to pose difficulties for many users.[1] Although users were able to develop an adequate working ability with system commands and search procedures fairly easily, they often found conceptualization of their information need, construction of search strategy, and selection of appropriate controlled vocabulary perplexing. More recently, Sewell and Teitelbaum noted the problems users have with explosions and subheadings.[2] In fact, research on online searching over the years has consistently shown that the major problems encountered by users are not with search procedures and commands, but with the problem solving and other conceptual aspects of the search process.[3] These problems do not affect only end users; many experienced searchers have similar difficulties. Recent advances in software design have made the procedural aspects of searching easier than ever, but have as yet contributed little towards ameliorating these problems.

Although there are considerable differences between the use of manual and electronic systems for information retrieval, many of the problems users encounter in the manual search process derive from the same sources. Conceptualization of the information need, development of an appropriate search strategy, and use of controlled vocabulary are more formidable obstacles to successful searching in manual tools than are the details of deciphering citations, interpreting catalog cards and call numbers, organization of indexes, or shelf arrangements. It was awareness that these and other topics of traditional library skills instruction were secondary to successful library use that served as the impetus for the change to bibliographic instruction in academic libraries. Whatever the inadequacies of bibliographic instruction in its current state, with its emphasis on generic search strategies and overgeneralized perspectives on structure of the literature, it has at least attempted to address the more difficult aspects of searching at a level appropriate to college freshmen and sophomores. Yet, even at colleges and universities with strong bibliographic instruction programs, approaches to instruction in the use of newer information retrieval sources have proven elusive. Online catalogs, CD-ROM devices, and online systems for end-user searching have renewed the challenge to improve instructional programs, to move beyond training in the use of these tools, to begin "mainstreaming" technology, and to develop educational programs that incorporate and build upon both the power of the technology and the insight it provides into information management. There are several obstacles that have, so far, thwarted rapid progress in this direction.

The first of these obstacles involves the immense impact technology has had, not only upon our practice and goals, but also upon our perception of the phenomena and processes that make up our working environment. The dominant world view in modern society is mechanical.[4] That which can be described in terms of cause and effect, or explained as a step-by-step, linear process, is accepted more readily as knowledge. That which cannot is suspect. As a result, there is a tendency to emphasize mechanics. Since almost everyone shares this world view, content that can be organized and presented in cause and effect or procedural terms is relatively easy to learn and easy to teach.[5] The mechanics and procedures of searching organized information sources, whether manual or electronic, are readily taught and learned through training. The strategic aspects of searching are more difficult to reduce to a mechanical level successfully, and the conceptual aspects of searching present even greater problems. These aspects of searching, which represent the areas in which users experience their greatest difficulties, often receive inadequate attention in training.

The second obstacle, and perhaps an explanation for the emphasis on the procedural at the expense of the conceptual, is a lack of understanding of the problem-solving processes that information retrieval and management entail. Flowcharts of the problem-solving processes of reference service, which may be similar to problem solving in information seeking, have been attempted.[6] Models of online search processes have been proposed.[7] Whatever insight these efforts may have provided, it is also evident that they do not adequately describe the processes; at most they offer a procedural skeleton. Research in cognitive science and computer simulation suggest that human problem-solving processes are much more complex than linear, procedural, step-by-step descriptions are capable of explaining.[8]

A third area for concern involves the differing perspectives inherent in professional cultures. Each discipline or realm of professional practice encourages distinct approaches to knowledge, learning, and problem solving. Just as lawyers, politicians, engineers, chemists, activists, and businessmen might all differ in their approaches to remedying the problem of toxic waste disposal, librarians and the diverse clientele they serve may differ considerably in their relationships to the literature and preferred methods for management of the literature. Although research has revealed some of these differences, there is a tendency for those within a particular professional culture to believe in the validity of their perspectives and approaches, and to assert the importance of their methods. Health sciences librarians have worked hard to try to adapt to, accommodate, and incorporate the relationships client groups hold with the literature. But there remains much to be learned before the differences between the culture of librarianship and the professional cultures of library clientele are really understood.

A part of the culture of any profession is the educational experience. Those within a profession pass along the knowledge of the discipline in ways that are believed to be effective, assuring continuity and perpetuating the knowledge base of the profession. But the ways of communication and education differ between the professions, of course, which complicates effective dissemination of knowledge across disciplinary lines. There is a tendency to communicate what is known in ways that are familiar within the profession. Educationally, there is a tendency to teach as one learned or as one has seen others teach. In library schools and in library practice, as in other disciplines and professions, formal instruction most often concentrates on facts, procedures, and tools. The conceptual aspects of professional practice, and effective problem solving, are more often learned experientially, either on the job or in simulated situations. As a result, it is difficult to convey this knowledge across disciplinary boundaries; and it is difficult to accommodate the preferred learning styles of those in other professional groups. This fosters an element of mystery to professional practice, as well as inevitable misunderstandings, however slight, of what professional practice involves. It also fosters a sense of self-sufficiency and "rightness" about practices within the profession which is perpetuated not only through the educational experience, but also through the structure and tools of practice. Consequently, it may be easier to instruct others about the characteristics and procedural aspects of the use of tools than it is to convey the conceptual aspects of their use and their place in the problem-solving and decision-making processes. Those within the profession find the nature and use of the tools obvious. Those viewing the tools from outside the profession do so from the perspective of their own professional culture, according to different value systems and anticipating different potential for application.

This leads to the final hurdle to be considered here: expectations. Any instructional effort is undertaken with expectations, not only about what is important for the learner to know, but also what the learner will do with that knowledge. And the learner enters an instructional opportunity with expectations about what knowledge is needed and how that knowledge might be applied. This is particularly true in instruction for adults intended to convey practical information. The discrepancies between that which librarians consider important to know and what should be the practical outcome of instruction, on the one hand, and what clientele consider important to know and what they see as the potential application, on the other, may be great. In teacher-guided instruction, the expectations of teachers are imposed upon the learner, and information is organized and conveyed in ways the teacher considers appropriate. This is the tradition of the educational system from grade school on. It was disaffection with teacher-guided instruction in recent decades that led to learner-guided instruction and open classroom approaches in some schools. The expectations of teachers about learning and instruction in these circumstances differ considerably from those of teachers involved in teacher-guided instruction. There is much to criticize in either approach, and many educators are seeking other alternatives. Library instructional efforts vacillate between the two. Formal instructional efforts tend to be teacher-guided, with the librarian deciding on content and controlling the classroom or learning process. Less formal efforts, such as one-on-one assistance, is more often learner-guided, with the librarian responding to the patron's immediate needs and providing advice about means of further progress. There are advantages and disadvantages with both approaches, and strong proponents of each. Most of the assumptions about the effectiveness of either approach, most of the expectations librarians have about learning styles of their clientele, and the compatibility of instructional methods with patrons' needs, are just that–assumptions. There has been little relevant research, especially in health sciences library settings, to guide instructional efforts or judge their effectiveness. Too often, expectations about clientele's needs and interests, and the appropriate methods for instruction, are based more on conjecture than knowledge; and assumptions about content and outcomes are too rarely questioned.

It has already been suggested that educational programs, in contrast to training efforts, focus more intently upon problem solving, decision making, and the conceptual aspects of information management. Developing such programs might seem unreasonable and, even perhaps, unnecessary in the light of the obstacles mentioned here: unreasonable due to the complexity of offering an educational experience that overcomes these problems in the brief time allotted the librarian under most instructional circumstances, and unnecessary because adult learners can best direct their learning and apply new knowledge according to their own proclivities. The difficulties users encounter in information management and exploitation of the tools available to them militates against this interpretation. Not only does research reveal the areas in which users have problems in online searching, for example, but it also suggests something about the inadequacies of training and the value of more educational emphasis in instruction. Users who receive only informal instruction, including one-on-one instruction from librarians, may find important gaps in their knowledge. The problems experienced by users who have received operational training in searching have already been touched upon. And those who receive advanced training may find that they search little better, but make more (and more sophisticated) errors. On the other hand, users who receive instruction with more emphasis on the conceptual aspects of searching, problem-solving processes, and development of search strategies have a more solid base for searching. Those who receive only operational training can usually perform basic searches, but those who receive instruction with a stronger educational emphasis can build upon their knowledge to improve their searching.

Instructional programs in libraries are often, by necessity, composed of relatively short sessions. Some libraries have successfully moved to seminar series or full courses. Unfortunately, even with the latter, content tends to be handled as discrete units, suggestive of individual training sessions, rather than an integrated educational program. The obstacles to developing educational programs in libraries are formidable, and probably preclude immediate moves toward full-scale educational programming. But lack of complete knowledge does not preclude incremental development. It would be difficult to turn a one- or two-hour training session in online searching into a full-fledged educational experience, but it could be made more educational by subordinating procedural and operational content and placing it within a context that emphasizes the conceptual and strategic aspects of searching. As more is learned about the problem-solving processes of library clientele, it may be possible to draw upon the decision-making processes of particular client groups to create more familiar contexts for learning. Clinicians, for example, might comprehend the searching and information management processes more readily if modelled after and presented in a context approximating the conceptual processes of diagnosis and case management. Laboratory researchers might respond more readily to models paralleling experimental methods. These and other approaches that bridge the gaps between professional cultures may improve our ability to communicate the nonprocedural aspects of effective information management. Opportunities to integrate information management into disciplinary curricula should enhance understanding of the instructional approaches most appropriate to client groups by providing insight into their expectations, learning styles, and educational milieu. Progress may be slow, and may involve more trial and error than might be wished, but educational programming in libraries is a realizable goal.

Progress toward educational programs in libraries will not be without its costs. The investment required to develop such programs, not only financially, but also administratively and professionally, will be considered in the next chapter.

REFERENCES

1. Lancaster, Frederick W. "Evaluation of On-Line Searching in MEDLARS (AIM-TWX) by Biomedical Practitioners." Urbana, IL: University of Illinois Graduate School of Library Science, 1972. (*Occasional Papers* #101); also ERIC ED 062 989).

2. Sewell, Winifred, and Teitelbaum, Sandra. "Observations of End User On-line Searching Behavior Over Eleven Years." *Journal of the American Society for Information Science* 37(July 1986):234-245.

3. Fenichel, Carol H. "The Process of Searching Online Bibliographic Databases: A Review of Research." *Library Research* 2(Summer 1980-81):107-127.

4. Rifkin, Jeremy. *Entropy; A New World View.* New York: Viking, 1980.

5. King, David N., and Baker, Betsy. "Teaching End Users To Search: Issues and Problems." In: Bungard, Teresa (ed.), *Bibliographic Instruction and Computer Database Searching.* Ann Arbor: Pierian, 1987.

6. Lancaster, Frederick W. *Measurement and Evaluation of Library Services.* Washington, DC: Information Resources Press, 1977, pp. 113-129.

7. Meadow, Charles T., and Cochrane, Pauline (Atherton), *Basics of Online Searching.* New York: John Wiley and Sons, 1981, pp. 133-142.

8. A nontechnical discussion of current thought on human problem solving, how it differs from computer information processing, and new attempts at computer modelling can be found in: Allman, William F. "Mindworks." *Science 86* 7(May 1986):22-31.

Chapter 3

Creating Educational Programs in Libraries: Part 3–Costs

David N. King

INTRODUCTION

This is the third chapter on information management education, and will complete an overview of some of the problems and issues surrounding the development of educational programs in libraries. The first in the series considered the distinction between training and education. Although the two overlap, training was described as a means of presenting learners with basic procedural knowledge which would enable them to perform practical tasks at an acceptable skill level. Education, on the other hand, was considered an effort aimed at offering learners a level of conceptual understanding conducive to continued development and problem solving. With instruction in MEDLINE searching as an example, it was suggested that training focuses on procedures, commands, system features, and terminological choices with the intent of providing users with the basics of search technique. Education lays a foundation of principles, for example, search strategy or conceptualizing information needs, with instruction in the use of a particular system serving as a means to higher ends. Information management education, then, if its intent were actually educational, would aim at mastery of the problem-solving processes of information management, rather than proficiency in the use of tools.

This chapter was first published in *Medical Reference Services Quarterly*, Vol. 7(1), 1988.

In the second chapter, some of the obstacles to development of educational programs in libraries were considered. The first was the mechanical world view which promotes a tendency to focus on the procedural aspects of systems (manual or electronic), as opposed to conceptual, process understanding. The second obstacle, which may derive from the first, involved a lack of understanding of the problem-solving processes that underlie information retrieval and management. The third consideration was the role of professional culture as a force that shapes perspectives and methods, and the importance of the differences between the professional culture of librarianship and that of library clientele. Fourth, the nature of the educational experience within a discipline, and the tendency to teach as one has learned, was seen as a factor complicating cross-disciplinary communication and instruction. And finally, the discrepancy between the expectations and intents of clientele, and those of librarians, was seen as an important aspect which can affect the effectiveness of any instructional effort. The result of these, and other more immediate limitations like the time available for instruction, have often led to instructional efforts that consist of various brief training sessions rather than educational programs.

In this, the third and last chapter, the costs of developing educational programs in health sciences libraries are addressed. These costs are not limited to budgetary considerations, but also include the professional and administrative investment required by the library and by librarians. These costs may exact a greater toll than can be accounted for in purely economic terms, but the benefits, if equally difficult to quantify, may exceed the expectations of librarians and clientele alike.

In discussing the costs of developing educational programs in libraries, all concerned must eventually look at the bottom line. The monetary costs of any library endeavor are unavoidable in the decision-making process, and especially so during periods of tightening budgets. Good administrators, and good department managers, attempt to allocate organizational resources on the basis of priorities, with greater emphasis on maintaining current services and programs at an acceptable level. Real innovation is usually placed further down the list of priorities, not only because of the effect innovative programs or services have on direct costs, but because the organizational costs associated with innovation involve much more than simply redistributing dollars. These other costs will, at some point, show up on the bottom line, but they cannot be considered exclusively within the context of budget. The development of educational programs in libraries, as opposed to training programs, involves organizational investments which transcend simple arithmetic. As with any innovative endeavor, decisions about whether or not to pursue major change in programming or service cannot be considered entirely in economic terms. It may be useful to look at the more familiar direct budgetary costs before taking up the issue of these other economic concerns.

INSTRUCTIONAL COSTS

The costs associated with instructional efforts in libraries are typically examined in terms of the direct cost of delivering the instructional product. Some of these direct costs appear in Table 3.1, which compares costs of courses offered by an information management education (IME) program and a library school. The IME class meets once a week over the 13-week term for one hour per meeting. The librarian, on average, spends about five hours of preparation time for each hour of class, and spends about four hours per class for follow-up activities such as grading and individual consultation. Due to the short class times and the inclusion of training in online searching outside class time, individual consultation and follow-up time with students is important. The librarian's time accounts for almost two-thirds of the total cost of the instruction program. Other costs include the time of support staff for preparation of graphics; typing and copying printed materials; directing stray students and other miscellaneous activities; about ten hours of online time for demonstrations and hands-on exercises; materials; and other expenses such as fringe benefits of those involved, equipment maintenance, and so on. Not included are costs of equipment purchase and installation, overhead, and other indirect costs.

For comparison, the cost of a library school medical reference course is presented. More hours are spent in class, but, proportionately, approximately the same number of hours are devoted to individual consultation. The total hours spent in preparation time and

TABLE 3.1. Some Direct Costs of a Semester Course

Costs	IME Course		Library School Course	
1. Staff time	Hours	Dollars	Hours	Dollars
a. Instructional				
Classroom hours	13		40	
Preparation time	65		120	
Follow-up activities	40		60	
Individual consulting	18		40	
TOTAL HOURS	136		260	
APPROXIMATE COST		$1,904*		$3,500**
b. Support staff time		$ 300		$ 400
2. Online services		150		350
3. Materials		100		250
4. Other (fringe benefits, etc.)		500		600
TOTAL COSTS (est.)		$2,954		$5,100

* Based on salary of $28,000 per calendar year (approx. $14 per hour)
** Based on salary of $28,000 per academic year (five-eighths time teaching)

follow-up activities is greater, but the number of hours per hour of class time is somewhat less. More than twice as much online time is provided students, and more materials are used in the course.

There are some major differences between a library school course and a credit IME course in terms of content, purpose, environmental and student characteristics, and expectations. A good IME course, for example, might include components on organizing personal reprint files and personal information management–topics that might only be covered in passing in a library school course. The latter might place greater emphasis on understanding the structure of the literature of various constituencies, their information-seeking proclivities, specialized services such as clinical medical librarian (CML) programs, and in-depth exploration of print and online tools, whereas these might receive less emphasis in an IME course. The purpose of a medical reference course is to prepare students for medical library practice, an unlikely goal for IME. And since library school courses are central to the professional goals of most students who enroll, expectations concerning the time and effort that students will invest in the course are much higher. In an IME course, the students might be willing to spend one or two hours of out-of-class time each week; library school students might find it necessary to spend eight to 12 hours.

The cost to students of an instructional program is rarely considered on the tally sheets. But it is often the investments made by students that determine the educational potential of an instructional effort. A library school course may require only slightly more time on the part of the teacher, but three to four times as much on the part of students. The variable quality of library school courses (or any other for that matter) is testimony to the fact that hours spent do not assure hours spent well, and some library school courses may be short of true educational experiences. Even so, the increased time offers the opportunity to move beyond basic training to education.

Given the circumstances, it is probably unrealistic to expect more from students taking IME courses than has been described. The cost to those who take the course may be too great if the time required of students is increased. After all, for most who take such a course as an elective, learning the basics of searching and personal file management are of interest, but not at the top of the list of priorities. Students may see little relationship between the content of the course and their professional careers. They may be perfectly satisfied with a basic training experience, and less interested in an educational one. Many are of the opinion that they can tell what they need to know, and demonstrate less patience with those who would tell them what they *ought* to know. And most of them are confident of their knowledge and their ability to master any task quickly, as need arises, given a brief introduction. Most are probably quite happy with effective training.

Developmental Program Costs

A few of the limitations of training were considered earlier. Most notable in this respect are research findings which suggest that learners are unable to develop adequate mental models without good conceptual models as a foundation. Those receiving training in online searching, for example, may be able to follow the step-by-step procedures and commands to perform searches at a basic level, but lack of a conceptual understanding of the search process and system use limits their ability to perform more sophisticated searches and limits their ability to improve their search skills. Moreover, instruction without a conceptual base forces learners to develop their own mental models, which may be quite erroneous and counterproductive. (It may be noted that research also suggests that many librarians and search intermediaries, in spite of years of searching experience, often search at a less-thansophisticated skill level. This could reasonably be attributed, at least in part, to the instruction they received: training.)[1-3]

In addition to the limitations of procedural training, there are further reasons why libraries should consider moving in the direction of educational service. First, many of the educational institutions served by health sciences libraries are reexamining their curricula, with an eye toward preparing their students for lifelong learning. Libraries can contribute significantly to educational efforts toward this end, if the right means and roles can be found. Second, there is good reason to believe that technological advances have precipitated a climate conducive to increased library participation in health sciences education and practice. Libraries can contribute significantly if they design the right services and educational "products" for their clientele. Finally, despite much early concern about resistance to change during the period of adopting and adapting to newer technologies in libraries, many libraries and many librarians are thriving in the evolving environment and enthusiastically pursuing the challenge of the new opportunities that surround them.

All the foregoing suggests that the time is ripe for educational efforts by libraries, and that a move toward more educationally sound instruction is needed. But, as was evident in Chapter 2, there are some formidable obstacles to be overcome. The cost of developing educational services in health sciences libraries is not easily accounted for in traditional budgeting and accounting. More is involved than simply offering more of the same sort of instruction, or simply expanding what is currently offered.

Before libraries can provide good educational service to their clientele, a solid knowledge base is required. Too little is, as yet, understood about the information management needs of clientele. Much of the research on information seeking and use among health professionals fails to focus on specific client groups or specific information needs and uses. It is accepted that the information needs of researchers, for example, will differ from those of clinicians. But there is little specific knowledge available. Do the information needs and habits of pediatricians differ from those of heart surgeons, and do those of general practitioners coincide with either? And unfortunately, what little research has accumulated predates the widespread availability of microcomputer applications for information access and management, and ready access to bibliographic database services. Much of what was known about the information-seeking and use patterns among health professionals is outdated.

Much has changed in respect to library practice in recent years as well. The knowledge, skills, and activities of librarians have been reshaped as the library has evolved. There is a need for better understanding of the areas in which librarians' expertise and client needs overlap. Much of the expertise available in libraries goes untapped because librarians do not know it is available or might be useful to them. There has been little systematic effort to identify the types of expertise currently available and new ways in which it might be applied.

More important, there has been little effort to systematically consider what is meant by information management, what knowledge and skills health professionals need to access and manage their information effectively, and what expertise librarians must have in order to meet the need. To offer training without such knowledge is one thing; to attempt real educational endeavors without such understanding is quite another, and probably folly. Even a cursory glance at past practice suggests that most instructional programming provided by libraries has derived from assumptions about what users ought to know, and has been limited in scope. Librarians can often guess correctly when the focus of instruction is aimed at use of the library and its tools. But educational efforts aimed at development of information-management knowledge and skills *should* derive more from the professional practices and needs of clientele, rather than those of librarians. And the more specific to the client group, the better the chance of success.

Basic understanding of principles of learning and teaching principles is needed.[4] Educational endeavors should be based on conscious decisions about the preferred learning styles of clientele, and the most effective ways of teaching. Because of the professional culture of librarianship and the tendency to teach as one learned, much instruction offered by libraries is founded on library practice and education. An educational effort for a client group, such as medical students, should more reasonably be founded in their professional education and practice. It has already been suggested that the principles be derived, not from the decision-making processes and practices of librarians, but from the decision-making processes and practices familiar to the client group. Even the practice of drawing parallels between print and online sources is questionable, since it may complicate matters by dealing with two unfamiliar tools rather than one. The more closely information-management principles and techniques can be tied to the principles and techniques of the professional group, the better the chance of offering a rewarding educational experience.

All these points concern the need for knowledge, and the cost of acquiring it will not be insignificant. It will require a dedicated effort, if not formal research, to build a knowledge base sufficient to serve as a foundation for information management education. It will require that librarians venture into the realm of their clientele to gain insight into their professional culture, their educational methods and learning styles, their decision-making processes, and their information needs and behavior. The librarian will have to be accepted outside the library in the process, and be able to contribute meaningfully to decisions made at a level beyond the internal affairs of the library. Certainly, the librarian will have to be an informed participant, an educator, and have excellent communication skills. Even more challenging is the fact that, given the importance of credentials in academic education, librarians in medical school settings may find the MLS inadequate to the role of educator.

The costs associated with the development of knowledge and expertise can be formidable, and difficult to quantify. Equally hard to account for are the administrative costs that are involved with developing educational services. An administrative stamp of approval to offer instruction will not go far. The library must be committed to becoming an active force in the education of its clientele, and must work toward an organizational structure and climate that facilitates that end. A new balance between the question-answering, document delivery tradition of information services, and the educational role of the library, must be struck. Organizational flexibility will be required in the process, along with effective management processes that will accommodate change. The venture into education will affect almost every other person and activity in the library. More than the monetary costs that might be incurred in personnel and management time is the risk involved in any innovative endeavor that affects staff and standard practices.

Finally, there are the costs associated with expansion of the professional role of librarians. Most instruction provided by libraries to date has not required that librarians move mentally outside the library. If the instruction has not been provided in the library, it typically involved only short excursions beyond the doors. The library remained "home base." In fact, since instruction has often been only one of several service activities, with time also given to providing reference and search services by many librarians involved in instruction, the role of instructor is often considered secondary. This will not be the case if information management education is to move beyond training. The librarian will find it necessary to adopt the role of educator. A good IME program will probably be integrated into the curriculum and into courses as part of the education of students. For residents, practitioners, researchers, and others, it will probably require a great deal of time in the professional settings of these groups. Instruction of the training sort may still be offered, though not necessarily in the library. In the early stages of development, the IME librarian may share some of the same patterns that CML librarians do. But as IME is integrated into curricular and client practice, the librarian may spend less and less time in the library, and may be involved in few other service activities. The price to be paid is a personal one, and only the individual can decide if the benefits outweigh the cost of redefining the professional role.

The rewards for developing educational programs in libraries are real, but difficult to quantify. Certainly, clientele will benefit from better ability to manage their information needs and resources. The library will benefit by becoming recognized as not only a warehouse for collections with helpful staff, but a center for expertise in information management. Closer ties to the institution served, better working relationships with departments and clientele who might not have been encountered otherwise, and librarians in client settings to increase visibility and promote the library, will place the library in a stronger position. From the moment the library begins to work toward developing educational programs by improving its knowledge of its clientele, it will be able to identify ways of enhancing other services. And the personal and professional growth of the librarians involved will be immeasurable.

Whether the benefits are worth the investment is a decision that can only be made by each library in its own way. But IME represents yet another opportunity for the library to take a leadership role in the development of health services and the health professions, and to shape the new future of health sciences libraries and health science librarianship.

NOTES

1. Bellardo, Trudi. "What Do We Really Know About Online Searchers?" *Online Review* 9(1985):223-239.

2. Fenichel, Carol H. "The Process of Searching Online Bibliographic Databases: A Review of Research." *Library Research* 2(1980-81):107-127.

3. Olroyd, B.K., and Citroen, C.L. "Study of Strategies Used in On-line Searching." *On-Line Review* 1(1977):293-310.

4. Wanger, Judith. "Education and Training for Online Systems." *Annual Review of Information Science and Technology* 14(1979):219-245.

Chapter 4

Administrative Structures for Education Programs

Francesca Allegri

INTRODUCTION

Discussions about the way to organize and manage an education program within a library usually result in three options: a librarian within the reference department is assigned responsibility for the program, a coordinator is appointed with authority to enlist the help of librarians throughout the organization, or a separate department is established to run the program. Two years ago, the staff of Information Management Education Services (IME) in the Health Sciences Library at the University of North Carolina at Chapel Hill discussed other options as part of a strategic planning effort underway at the library. Nine possible models came out of a series of brainstorming sessions. These are outlined below with the advantages and disadvantages of each structure as viewed from the IME department setting. Major considerations underlying these models were the level of visibility that the model would provide to education, whether staff would be shared with other departments, and where leadership for educational programs would reside. The models are not listed in any particular order.

POSSIBLE MODELS

A separate department with a department head reporting to the library director was the model in place at the Health Sciences Li-

This chapter was first published in *Medical Reference Services Quarterly*, Vol. 10(2), Summer 1991

brary at the time of the discussions described above. The following were viewed to be the advantages and disadvantages of this model.

Advantages:
- demonstrates commitment to education;
- gives internal status to the program;
- enables high visibility; national as well as local and regional presence were achieved rapidly with this model;
- provides a dedicated advocate (department head) for education programs;
- guarantees participation/input into major library-wide decisions;
- provides better communication between IME staff and rest of the library staff and administration;
- provides a resource person (department head) who is actually involved in the programs;
- removes competition for the department head's time;
- enables staff to develop and improve teaching skills;
- enables higher level of quality control of support materials;
- provides continuity with schools and departments outside the library;
- enables offering a higher volume and greater variety of programs;
- enhances continuity within the IME programs; ensures the teaching staff are genuinely interested in education;
- improves ability to adapt to the rhythm of the school year;
- removes conflict for time between project planning and on-demand services, thus keeping the priority for education high.

Disadvantages:
- increases the number of department heads;
- makes recruiting more difficult because positions are specialized;
- makes cross-training with reference and computing services necessary;
- costs more to have a department head and staff with special expertise, equipment, and space;
- can only be implemented in larger libraries;

– may reduce flexibility in scheduling because staff have specialized roles.

A second model would be the same as the first except that a coordinator would head the unit and report to a department head.

Advantages:
- same as the first model as they pertain to a staff dedicated to education;
- costs less for a coordinator than a department head;
- potential is better for cross-over knowledge being shared with the department in which the education unit is located.

Disadvantages:
- potential exists for conflicts of interest on the part of the department head;
- dilutes the education perspective;
- conveys less status, visibility, and commitment to education;
- coordinator lacks direct participation in the management team;
- department head may not be agreeable to or understand the education planning mode.

A third model follows the lines of the two above except that there is no coordinator; the education unit reports directly to the department head who serves as coordinator.

Advantages:
- same as the first model as they pertain to a staff dedicated to education;
- costs even less than the first two models.

Disadvantages:
- same as in the second model, only exaggerated;
- the department head has a heavier workload and more competition for resources;
- lack of a dedicated coordinator may adversely affect recruiting.

A fourth model would combine education completely with an existing department; responsibility for education would be shared.

Advantages:
- personnel costs are less than for the previously discussed models;
- cross-over knowledge is potentially good;
- if combined with reference, exposure to certain types of user questions is greater, facilitating instruction pertaining to those areas.

Disadvantages:
- the flip side of the first model's advantages of having a dedicated staff, e.g., lack of expertise/interest on the part of some instructors;
- could result in a decrease in the type of programs offered;
- staff must deal with conflicting tasks;
- same disadvantages as the second and third models;
- department head assumes all responsibility for administration, expertise, and resources;
- removes a career ladder step, i.e., from reference to specialization in education.

A fifth model would combine education with another department while maintaining a coordinator but not a dedicated staff. This is one of the most common models in place at the present time.

Advantages:
- some administrative tasks are assumed by the coordinator;
- personnel costs are less than those models with a dedicated staff;
- other advantages are the same as for the fourth model.

Disadvantages:
- the coordinator must recruit and train teachers while dealing with the disadvantages of model four, particularly a staff with other tasks demanding attention;
- leaves little time for planning and preparation of teaching material.

A sixth model is to have a department head for education who has the responsibility and authority to contract with other departments in the library for projects and hours.

Advantages:
- works better for workshops and orientations;
- helps in obtaining good subject expertise of instructors;
- easily allows scaling back on education programs.

Disadvantages:
- difficult to use this model with course-related or credit courses in which continuity and duplication are issues;
- poses a staff development problem if instructors lack teaching skills;
- it is difficult to obtain and maintain instructors' commitment to non-primary functions;
- increases the number of department heads with a one-person department;
- increases the difficulty of recruiting for the department head position;
- increases the difficulty of starting new programs;
- may necessitate hiring more staff in other departments.

A seventh model is to only provide one-on-one instruction, i.e., to have no education department or programs.

Advantages:
- costs little if there is no commitment to build up the reference staff;
- user receives instruction at the time of expressed need, depending on the reference staff's availability.

Disadvantages:
- does not meet significant demand for group instruction;
- the library may not have the option of referring requests for group instruction to other libraries;
- not cost-effective on the part of the reference staff, i.e., much effort is duplicated;
- counter to trends in medical librarianship.

An eighth model consists of centralizing leadership for education programs in the library but recruiting instructors from outside the library.

Advantages:
- personnel costs are kept inexpensive;
- strengthens potential of having instructors with subject expertise;
- potentially broadens the visibility for the program;
- increases credibility of instructors with the audience as content pertains to their discipline;
- builds a pool of more "educated" users who could serve as library advocates on other occasions.

Disadvantages:
- introduces lack of control/autonomy of the library's programs;
- instructors may lack commitment to the library; the rate of turnover of instructors may increase;
- difficult to recruit for instructors because of their time constraints and the lower rewards for teaching at many institutions;
- introduces the possibility of lack of teaching expertise, knowledge, and understanding of the library;
- makes educational follow-up more difficult;
- increases difficulties of communicating with instructors;
- increases difficulty of recruiting an education coordinator;
- may complicate support issues, e.g., materials development, printing, use of equipment and space;
- introduces "training the trainers" issues, e.g., dilution of library knowledge, scheduling, back-up.

The ninth, and final, model consists of elevating education to an "umbrella" department, encompassing such functions as reference, online services, consultation services, and microcomputer services.

Advantages:
- implies the strongest emphasis on education of the models described here;
- increases likelihood that other library services will be viewed from an educational perspective;
- has the same advantages as merging education with other departments.

Disadvantages:
- has the same disadvantages of merging education with other departments;
- may be too large to manage as one department;
- microcomputer user support or other functions may be too different to combine with education or reference.

CONCLUSION

The above is, by no means, an exhaustive list of models or of advantages and disadvantages. Those who have actually used one or more of these models will see added benefits and drawbacks of them. In addition, some of these pluses and minuses need to be examined from a different library's perspective. However, it is hoped that these may spark some new thoughts on arrangements for providing educational services.

Chapter 5

Developing a Teaching Effectiveness Program for Librarians: The Ohio State University Experience

Virginia Tiefel

How does a large university library with limited financial resources and staff meet the needs of its librarians to develop and sustain effective teaching skills in a burgeoning library user education program? How can their needs be identified and a program developed to meet them? Can such a program be replicated at other institutions? The Ohio State University Libraries have made substantial progress in mounting a teaching effectiveness program, and it is believed that the structure and much of the content of the program are transferable.

At the Ohio State University, there exists a very strong commitment to the concept of teaching information skills, not only on the part of the library faculty and staff, but also on the part of the Libraries' and University's senior administrators. In addressing a faculty/library colloquium in 1982, Edward H. Jennings, President of the Ohio State University observed:

> We're all aware that we are in an age of information explosion—not only of information in specific disciplines, but also in the need for access to knowledge that cuts across—and combines and uses knowledge from—various fields. It must be the mission of the University and of all of our faculty to help

This chapter was first published in *Medical Reference Services Quarterly*, Vol. 7(4), 1988.

43

develop those critical abilities of information usage in all of our students.

In 1986 the Ohio State University Libraries (OSU) developed a strategic planning document for the future of the library system which expressed this philosophy about library instruction:

> To be useful citizens of an information-dependent society, students must be taught how to identify, locate, evaluate, and utilize information in an effective manner. . . . In addition to providing instruction in traditional bibliography and basic library use techniques, librarians are also responsible for an ever-larger role in teaching the use of new information technology.

Given the emphasis on teaching information skills to students at Ohio State and renewed attention to improving teaching, generally, on the campus and nationally, some concerted effort to improve the quality of library instruction was seen to be essential. Indeed, this concern has been expressed by many librarians in the profession. The editors of a recent book on teaching librarians stated their purpose was "to address the need for a continuing program designed to enhance and update the teaching skills needed for providing effective instruction to the students who use the library."[1]

THE NEED AT THE OHIO STATE UNIVERSITY LIBRARIES

The library user education program at OSU was formally established in 1978. The program now reaches approximately 20,000 students every year with some form of course-related instruction. As the program has developed, the number of librarians teaching in it has increased proportionately. With every member of the library faculty expected to participate in some aspect of library user education, many librarians expressed a desire/need to improve their teaching skills. In addition, the Libraries' freshman instruction program, which relies very heavily on the contributions of volunteer librarians, was manifesting the need for more effective teaching.

This became apparent in comments by both librarians and freshman instructors who had observed some student inattention during the library presentation.

In its initial response to these expressed and perceived needs, the library user education office sponsored an ad hoc "communications workshop" and a full-day teaching workshop in the early 1980s, both conducted by OSU departmental faculty. In 1984, a national leader in library instruction was brought in for a day-long workshop that dealt with both theoretical and practical issues. While these activities were enthusiastically received by the librarians who attended, evaluations clearly reflected the need for an ongoing teaching program.

Three surveys of the library faculty conducted between 1979 and 1984 revealed their primary concerns about user education to be the development and strengthening of teaching techniques and assistance in working with classroom faculty. In the area of teaching techniques, librarians wanted to know more about how to plan instruction generally, organize lectures, write instructional objectives, motivate students, begin an instruction program, develop materials, and handle large classes. They wanted to learn more about how to apply psychological principles of learning and use techniques that would help them to work effectively with classroom faculty. They wanted to discuss innovative approaches to instruction and their acceptability to others and have opportunities to share experiences and exchange ideas. A more recent evaluation done in conjunction with two videotaping workshops in summer 1986 showed the same priorities: how to develop teaching techniques, evaluate instruction in terms of goals and objectives, plan lessons, create materials, involve students, and teach large classes.

PLANNING THE PROGRAM

In the mid-1980s, with the need for an ongoing, comprehensive teaching effectiveness program clearly established, expertise to help in the planning and development of such a program was sought. A teaching consultant from the campus' Center for Teaching Excellence (CTE) worked with librarians over a period of months to develop instructional goals and objectives and program activities. Librarians wrote the instructional goals and objectives and the teaching consultant developed the program activities which would offer a variety of approaches to achieve instructional objectives. Organized into five learning concepts, activities were applied to instructional objectives. For example, to orient librarians to the user education program, a handbook of policies and procedures would be written and a mentoring system established. At the next level of building learning skills, handouts and workshops are appropriate modes of instruction. The activities would be initiated where applicable to achieve the instructional objectives.

The following is a list of the instructional goals and objectives developed by the OSU librarians.

Instructional Goals:

   A. Librarians will become more effective teachers and communicators.
   B. Librarians will become more confident about their teaching abilities.

Instructional Objectives:

   A. Librarians know and understand basic teaching/learning theory.
   B. Librarians know how to apply basic teaching techniques.
   C. Librarians are able to develop a lesson plan.
   D. Librarians are able to evaluate classroom presentations and materials.
   E. Librarians are able to prepare and present effective lectures.
   F. Librarians apply good communication skills in their teaching.
   G. Librarians make good use of audiovisual materials.

To achieve these objectives, the following program goals and activities were written by Dr. Nancy Chism, Center for Teaching Excellence, the Ohio State University.

Program Goals:

The program enables librarians to be more effective in their teaching.

Program Activities:

A. Orientation
   1. Handbook of policies and procedures
   2. Introductions/networking/mentoring
   3. Resource displays/information/tours
   4. Talks by experienced leaders

B. Skill-building
   1. Workshop
   2. One-on-one demonstration/practice
   3. Handouts/reading
   4. Demonstration films, etc.
   5. Observation of other teachers

C. Self-awareness
   1. Videotape feedback
   2. Small group instructional diagnosis
   3. In-class feedback devices
   4. Written instruments
   5. Peer visits

D. Understanding
   1. Inquiry/development projects
   2. Reading
   3. Consultation

E. Dialogue
   1. Conversation groups
   2. Lectures/seminars
   3. Conferences

The program was designed to address the needs of both new and experienced library faculty. Clearly, librarians new to OSU and/or to teaching needed an orientation to the library user education program and to teaching. They also needed help in developing their presentational skills, preferably in settings that provided practice and feedback. Experienced librarians especially wanted to know more about teaching techniques, planning lessons, and evaluation.

Activities based on the identified needs and instructional objectives were planned for each year, beginning in 1987.

IMPLEMENTING THE PROGRAM

A workshop for new library faculty was held in spring 1987 to introduce them to the user education program and office and to describe the various ways in which they could participate. It featured a panel discussion by librarians in the user education office and the Undergraduate Library, who described the program's history and development, instructional support provided by the office, and specific examples of opportunities for them to participate in instruction, such as workshops, research clinics, course-related instruction programs, and user education committee service. The ten librarian-attendees were given an evaluation form on which they were asked to list special skills, indicate in which activities they would like to participate, and offer suggestions for future workshops. The general comments and reactions were very positive.

Videotaping sessions were offered for new library faculty and any librarians who were new to teaching. Prior to the workshop the 12 participants were given materials on how to prepare effective presentations and asked to prepare a ten-minute presentation. They were videotaped in small groups, and the tapes played back for critique by the group. Discussion was led by the CTE teaching consultant. Evaluations of the workshops elicited two common responses. One was that the experience overall had been very positive and had increased individuals' confidence in their ability to teach. The other response was a recommendation that a continuing videotaping program be developed so that an individual could be videotaped intermittently over a period of time to monitor improvement.

The CTE teaching consultant then led a workshop in late spring 1987 in which teaching librarians shared their experiences. Titled "Triumphs and Tragedies," the workshop featured a lively discussion in which librarians identified their major concerns. Again, these included questions about how to motivate students, teach large classes, keep lectures to a reasonable length, make single lectures more effective, and reduce lecture time by incorporating more "hands on" teaching. In the discussion, the consultant emphasized three concepts:

1. We learn to teach by teaching.
2. Teaching is experiential.
3. We need to adapt our teaching to the learner.

No "breakthrough solutions" were uncovered, but possible approaches were offered and many of the issues and problems brought out in this forum were covered in an instructional planning workshop offered later in the summer. Librarian-participants unanimously agreed that the one hour allotted for the discussion workshop was inadequate.

The last workshop, which focused on how to plan for instruction, addressed the design of an instructional session, selection of content, and choice of appropriate delivery modes. The CTE teaching consultant again planned and led the workshop. After a general discussion, the group of 20 librarians was divided into four sections. Each group was given a real library teaching situation and asked to establish planning guidelines and plan an instruction session. The entire group then reconvened and shared the results of their planning. The attendees were enthusiastic in their evaluations of the workshop, with several recommending that the length of the next workshop be extended from an hour and a half to at least two hours.

COMMENT

Evaluations of the OSU Libraries' efforts to improve the teaching effectiveness of librarians, as has been stated, were very positive, even enthusiastic. The comments of participants in seven programs over the last two years were consistent in the concerns and recommendations expressed, the same topics recurring in suggestions for future workshops. Main concerns continue to be how to motivate students, improve lectures, apply the principles of instructional design and evaluation, write goals and objectives, and create materials. Recommendations included expansion of the videotaping workshop program and increasing the length of workshops. The participants invited more critical evaluation of their presentation skills and indicated a strong desire to meet to discuss experiences. An increased awareness of teaching and coping with its complexities was apparent in virtually all evaluations, as were expressions of increased confidence in the ability to teach effectively.

There were, in fact, few problems of any kind associated with the development of the program. The direct costs of the workshops were minimal. The services of neither the teaching consultant nor the videotaping laboratory were charged to the Libraries. Most of the handouts, required by all the workshops, were provided by the consultant and duplicated by the Libraries. The key ingredient of support was provided by both the library administration and individual library faculty. The Center for Teaching Excellence was critical to the success of these offerings in providing the expertise of an extremely knowledgeable and capable teacher.

THE FUTURE

Six activities are planned for 1988. The first is a lecture in the spring on motivating students, to be sponsored by CTE for faculty from throughout the University. Librarians will be urged to attend the lecture and a follow-up session for librarians to discuss applications of the lecture to library instruction will be offered. One or two videotaping sessions will be held in the summer. Since approximately one-third of the 90 library faculty have participated in this program in the last two years, librarians will be encouraged to repeat the experience for enrichment and reinforcement of past experience. Later in the summer, one workshop for librarians will focus on how to motivate and involve students, and another will examine how to evaluate an individual teaching session. A third workshop will provide a forum for librarians to share their experiences and ideas. The length of the workshops will be extended to two hours or more. All activities will be evaluated, and planning for a 1989 program will be based on the results of the evaluations.

Other activities planned include a topical workshop on writing and presenting research papers which will be offered in late spring 1988. It will be conducted by a faculty member in the Communication Department. Although that topic is outside the realm of the user education office's responsibility, the office has assisted in its planning in response to evaluation requests from library faculty. In an attempt to use print as well as workshop methods, a member of the office team will write an article on how to handle student questions in class. This will be published in the Libraries' internal user education newsletter.

APPLICATION TO OTHER LIBRARIES

The approach used in developing the OSU program is clearly applicable to other institutions. One must begin by determining what librarians perceive to be their needs and then enlist the help of those in or near the institution with expertise in addressing those needs. Many colleges or universities may not have a unit as structured or developed as Ohio State's Center for Teaching Excellence, but almost all campuses have faculty members who possess expertise in such areas as communication, evaluation, and teaching. Having identified the need and the expertise, one can plan an ongoing program based on established goals and objectives and incorporating proven methods of teaching and evaluation.

If library administrative support is not forthcoming, a strong case for such a program can be made by describing its obvious benefits in enabling librarians to be more effective and efficient in their teaching. A teaching effectiveness program can also favorably impress nonlibrary administrators and faculty who recognize that such a program can make a significant contribution to academic excellence.

NOTE

1. Clark, Alice S., and Jones, Kay F. *Teaching Librarians to Teach.* Metuchen, NJ: Scarecrow, 1986, p. viii.

Chapter 6

Defining What Instructional Librarians Need to Know About Information Technologies

Craig Mulder
Beth Layton

The mission of the Education Program at the Welch Medical Library is to foster effective scientific communication through education and practical application of information technologies at the Johns Hopkins Medical Institutions. To accomplish that mission, the Education Program offers general classes to the entire Hopkins community, as well as classes designed for specific departments and for integration within the curricula of the Schools of Medicine and Nursing. Another important component of the program is consulting with clients or small groups about information technologies. Instructors work with faculty, researchers, and students to integrate information technologies into their work.

In Fiscal Year 1991/92, the education program offered 360 educational activities with nearly 3200 people attending (see Table 6.1).

Instructors in the program cover a wide range of topics: information retrieval, information management, scientific writing, and computer training. They deal with reprint file management software, the online catalog, bibliographic and full-text databases, search interfaces, electronic mail, the Internet, file transfer, and telecommunications. Applications on the Macintosh, DOS, and UNIX platforms are supported.

This chapter was first published in *Medical Reference Services Quarterly*, Vol. 13(1), Spring 1994.

TABLE 6.1. Welch Education Program FY 1991/1992

	Classes	Attendees
Library Instruction	145	794
Personal Information Management	48	378
Curriculum-Based	16	254
Tours	n/a	154
Computer Training	104	642
Scientific Writing	18	818
Staff Training	29	157
TOTALS	360	3197

In order to provide assistance in all of these areas, instructors must be competent in relevant technologies. Given the diversity of the Hopkins environment, it is not possible for one person to know all the software or information tools used at our medical institutions. At best, an instructor becomes a "jack of all trades" and a master of none.

However, there is a strong need to keep the education staff, as a group, qualified to work in all of these areas and abreast of new developments. The following strategy helps meet that goal:

Step 1. Define the functions of the education program.

Step 2. For each function, determine the knowledge and skills required.

Step 3. For each skill, determine the tools needed and identify the local applications.

Step 4. For each tool, determine the necessary competencies. For each competency, determine whether all instructors need it or whether it should be assigned to one person.

Step 5. Use the competency matrix to audit each instructor's skills.

Step 6. For areas of deficiency, suggest options for staff training.

THE STRATEGY

Step 1. Define the Functions of the Education Program

To function effectively, instructors require knowledge and skills related to information technology. There are various ways by which to determine these requirements. One method is to consider the functions that are performed by each instructor and the type of knowledge required for each function. Another approach is to analyze the specific tasks performed by instructors and then derive a list of skills and types of knowledge. The potential problem with that approach is the likelihood of overlooking tasks that are not regularly or currently performed.

Education librarians at Welch are involved in three main functions:

- program management–librarians develop, evaluate, and market programs and manage staff, space, and money.
- activity management–librarians develop and evaluate instructional sessions and instructional tools.
- teaching and consulting–librarians teach the skills and tools required for scientific communication.

Step 2. Determine Required Knowledge and Skills

Scientific communication is the knowledge area of the teaching and consulting function (see Figure 6.1).

Step 3. Determine Needed Tools and Local Applications

For some skills, no computer-based tools are used. For instance, Welch instructors do not use a software application to perform the needs analysis skill.

Rather than describing the tools and applications used for each of the skills listed above, reprint management is used as an example (see Figure 6.2).

Step 4. Determine the Needed Competencies

The next step is to define the competencies required both for the general category and for specific applications. Each competency is

FIGURE 6.1. Functions, Knowledge, and Skills

Functions	Knowledge	Skills
Program Management	Development Evaluation	Project planning Basic stats, recording and analysis of data Reports, presenting data
	Marketing	Publicity Needs analysis
	Resource management	Electronic classroom design Budgeting Scheduling
Activity Management	Development Evaluation	Preparing classes and presentations
Teaching and Consulting	Scientific communication	Reprint management Using the library Information retrieval Communication, networking Scientific writing Knowledge, data management

examined and the required skill level needed for the education program and the individuals is set. For example, for the skill of generating bibliographies with Pro-Cite, it is important to decide whether each education librarian needs to know the skill or whether only one or two librarians in the department need to know it. This method helps to clarify the program's needs and to establish the skills for which each staff member is responsible.

The Welch Library has been working with faculty, researchers, support staff, and students in the area of reprint file management for more than six years. Instructors recommend to clients which package they should get to help them manage bibliographic information and create bibliographies. Instructors provide both formal classes in EndNote and Reference Manager, and individual help with other packages. General competencies are defined for all instructors:

- Comparability of locally supported applications
- Knowledge of the functions of bibliographic database with other text management software
- Understanding the mechanics of importing references

One instructor serves as an expert for each software system that is supported, with the understanding that everyone will be able to answer basic questions for all the software formally supported. Basic questions include those about importing from local databases, keyboard entry of references, retrieving references, and using on-line help (see Table 6.2).

Step 5. Audit Each Instructor's Skills

The "one" competencies are assigned to specific instructors by the program coordinator. This assignment ensures that all the necessary competencies are covered within the instructional program. Then each instructor must assess his or her own competencies based on the assignment by the program coordinator plus the "All" competencies listed in the matrix.

Step 6. Suggest Various Options for Staff Training

Once the audit is completed, staff members are responsible for developing their own professional development program. There are many options available. Tutorials are often available for specific

FIGURE 6.2. Skills, Tools, and Local Applications

Skills	Tools	Applications supported by Welch Instructors
Reprint Management	Work processing	WordPerfect® Microsoft Word
	Bibliographic database software	Reference Manager® EndNote® ProCite®

TABLE 6.2. Software Specific Competencies

Software Specific Competencies	EndNote Macintosh	EndNote DOS	Reference Manager Macintosh	Reference Manager DOS	Pro-Cite
Downloading and importing information	All	All	All	All	All
Installation	one	one	one	one	one
Importing references	All	All	All	All	All
Keyboard entry of references	All	All	All	All	All
Retrieval	All	All	All	All	All
Bibliography generation	one	one	one	one	one
Modifying bibliographic styles	one	one	one	one	one
Database management	one	one	one	one	one
Use of online help	All	All	All	All	All
Special features	one	one	one	one	one
Use of authority files	one	one	one	one	one
Contamination of database	one	one	one	one	one

programs and may be a part of the actual program. Good old hard copy items–books and journal articles–may be helpful. Audiovisual training such as computer-assisted instruction, audiotapes, or video-tapes may be purchased. For instance, there is a computer-assisted instruction tape set on File Maker Pro. The interactive "Navigating the Internet" tutorial accessed through the Internet had an enroll-ment of over 15,000. Local options include in-library staff training and institutional training programs. Professional organizations such as the Medical Library Association, Special Libraries Association, and American Library Association often provide useful sessions. The MEDLIB and BI-L listserves "advertise" sessions that may be appropriate. Commercial organizations also provide technology-based sessions.

In some areas, the entire staff may need additional training. In those cases, department-wide training is offered. One example is the Welch library's information technology seminar series. The current series is scheduled biweekly and covers areas such as file transfer, modems, ISDN, tcp/ip communications, and UNIX file structure.

CONCLUSION

This strategy of six steps can be used to determine the information technology skills and knowledge required by a department, and to assess staff education needs. This process offers a logical approach to analyzing staff education needs and provides a mechanism for addressing those needs more systematically.

Chapter 7

Breaking New Ground
in Curriculum Integrated Instruction

Rochelle L. Minchow
Kathryn Pudlock
Barbara Lucas
Stephen Clancy

INTRODUCTION

It is evident from numerous articles, reports, and conferences that information management is a new direction in medical education. Two benchmark publications have been key to shaping this new trend. The first publication is the now famous General Professional Education for Physicians (GPEP) Report, "Physicians for the Twenty-First Century." Among its salient highlights, the one most often cited is the need for medical faculties to offer educational experiences that require students to be active, independent learners and problem solvers, rather than passive recipients of information.[1] The second publication, *Medical Education in the Information Age: Proceedings of the Symposium on Medical Informatics,* discusses the necessity for medical schools to de-emphasize the mere acquisition of knowledge and emphasize information-organizing and problem-solving skills.

In response, medical schools are attempting to implement these strategies through the application of new techniques in information technology to teach medical students information-seeking skills rather than the rote memorization of a growing body of facts. These skills must go beyond the mere identification of major texts or specialty journals, but should encompass the structure and orga-

This chapter was first published in *Medical Reference Services Quarterly,* Vol. 12(2), Summer 1993.

nization of knowledge and the clinical and research decision process.[2] Accordingly, a new arena of medical education has developed in which health sciences librarians are playing integral roles. The librarians are assuming responsibility for instructing students and consulting with faculty on information management issues.[3]

COURSE-INTEGRATED INSTRUCTION

As a result of these trends, the University of California, Irvine (UCI) Biomedical Library took a proactive role to form a partnership between the Library and the College of Medicine. It was apparent from medical student questions at times of assignments that medical students had little knowledge in the utilization of the resources of the library. Yet information management classes have been offered on a weekly basis for the past six years as well as by appointment upon request, and medical students have not attended. During the times assistance has been provided to medical students, the librarians inquired into the reasons classes were not well received. Verbal responses primarily cited the lack of requirement and relevancy until needs arose. For these reasons, the librarians determined that the courses should be both required and attached to relevant needs, that is, integrated into the curriculum. With the cooperation of the College of Medicine, a survey was administered in September 1991 to 92 incoming medical students during their initial orientation. This survey was given to ascertain their interest in information-management skills and whether they felt these classes should be integrated into the curriculum. The results of the survey indicated a keen interest in the use of microcomputers, techniques to evaluate the literature critically, and database searching; and it especially highlighted that information management should be integrated within the curriculum, not offered as separate classes.

LITERATURE REVIEW

To support this need, an exhaustive review of the literature was conducted to investigate how information-management skills have been incorporated into medical school curricula. Although numerous databases were searched from 1980 to the present, the MEDLINE literature yielded the most relevant articles pertaining to collaborative efforts between medical schools and health sciences libraries which met the criteria for integrated instruction as defined by Allegri, i.e., faculty outside the library are involved in the design, execution, and evaluation of the program; the instruction is directly related to the students' course work and/or assignments; students are required to participate; and the students' work is graded or credit is received for participation.[4]

The University of Illinois College of Medicine,[5,6] the University of North Carolina at Chapel Hill,[7] the University of Tennessee College of Medicine,[8] Wright State University School of Medicine,[9] Mount Sinai School of Medicine of the City University of New York,[10] the University of Texas Medical School at Houston,[11] and the University of Missouri-Kansas City School of Medicine[12] all chose to incorporate library instruction in conjunction with clinical clerkships. Other schools have integrated library instruction into the medical school curriculum through content courses,[13,14] elective courses,[15] or seminars.[16,17]

There is tremendous variety in the content and the sources used to teach information-management skills. Core skills taught included the organization of biomedical literature; MeSH, printed indexes, and abstracting tools; printed sources, i.e., dictionaries, textbooks; style manuals; and general search strategy development.

All of the programs taught independent online searching skills as a means of keeping abreast of the current literature. These skills included coverage of computerized systems offering health sciences databases. The appropriateness of online versus printed sources; selection of appropriate databases; Boolean logic; MeSH and advanced search techniques were computer skills covered.

Critical appraisal, research design, current awareness, and personal file management were more advanced skills offered by the University of Illinois, the University of Tennessee College of Medicine, and the University of Minnesota.

Integration of library management skills into the medical curriculum proved successful in all programs. Student evaluations were positive and indicated that the instruction was a valuable tool during their course of study. Burrows,[14] Frasca,[6] Dorsch,[5] Proud,[13] and Graves[8] concluded that integrating information skills instruction into content courses in the medical school curriculum and designing active learning opportunities for this instruction are effective and efficient approaches to implementing many of the recommendations of the *GPEP Report.* Additionally, Burrows notes that these basic skills are reinforced and built upon in subsequent years throughout the medical curriculum. Learning these skills is reinforced by presenting and using them at the time of need or "teachable moment" rather than in the abstract.[18] The strategy also enhances the content of the primary curriculum and those cognitive skills generally considered to be central to graduate level education: concept learning, problem solving, and critical thinking.

A NEW APPROACH
TO COURSE-INTEGRATED INSTRUCTION

Armed with successful models discussed in the literature coupled with the survey results, a presentation was given to the Council of Course Coordinators and the Curriculum and Educational Policy Committee of the College of Medicine to promote the integration of instruction at UC Irvine. Concurrently, the College of Medicine expressed an interest in initiating problem-based learning (PBL). As defined by Barrows,

> Problem-based learning, properly designed, will allow students to integrate, use, and reuse newly learned information in the context of the patients' problems; the symptoms, signs, laboratory data, course of illness, etc., provide the cues for retrieval in the clinical context.[19]

PBL has several tenets which were compatible with the College of Medicine's educational goals.

> A primary educational aim of problem-based learning (PBL) is to teach problem-solving skills. The underlying premises, supported by research, are that problem-solving skills can be learned or enhanced and these skills are essential to good clinical judgement. A second educational aim is to integrate the basic sciences with the clinical sciences throughout the

curriculum. This integration helps students see the relevance of the basic sciences to clinical medicine and also establishes a tangible clinical base from which to retain the knowledge. A third educational aim is to develop lifelong learners, a commitment required of today's physician. The problem-based educational setting promotes active, independent learning and thus is believed to nurture lifelong learning habits.[20]

With the goal of information skills instruction to promote active, independent learning, this proved an opportune time to combine teaching information skills within the context of problem-based learning. A further evaluation of the literature demonstrated a paucity of experiences with PBL and health sciences library skills integration. Only one article proved pertinent in the analysis of the impact on the library of problem-based learning.[20] As of this writing, there are no reports where the librarians are involved in the actual implementation of a PBL program between faculty and students or where librarians also provided guided assistance through the literature assignments.

A five-week summer course served as a pilot for this new approach to medical education. Labeled "Preparation and Readiness for the Zenith in Education" (PRIZE), this program was offered to fifteen second-year minority medical students, or approximately two-thirds of the minority students in the second-year class. These students volunteered to participate in this pilot problem-based program to prepare for the United States Medical Licensing Examination (USMLE), as well as for the second year of medical school. During the introductory week, a traditional lecture was presented by the faculty consisting of basic information on pathology and pharmacology and the techniques of taking a medical history. A series of four clinical problems using a problem-based approach was the focus of the program. Each problem was presented as a typical clinical case by a faculty member and as a problem-solving session facilitated by two to three fourth-year medical students. Appendix A illustrates a representative case on lymphoma. In addition, a section on the use of library resources was presented by four reference librarians. The goal of the library instruction was to assist the students in becoming active, independent users of the library. The objectives were kept to a minimum as only a total of four hours was allotted for the formal component of library instruction. The objectives were: (1) to provide an understanding of the organization of biomedical literature; (2) to provide instruction on search strategy and selection of appropriate sources, i.e., print vs. online; (3) to review the University of California's MELVYL[R]* CATALOG; and (4) to provide instruction in MELVYL[R] MEDLINE[R]** including the use of Boolean logic, Medical Subject Headings (MeSH), and advanced searching techniques, e.g., subheadings, explosions, limiting.

The library instruction was held in the Learning Resource Center (LRC) in the Biomedical Library. The LRC contains sixteen computer terminals connected to the campus fiber-optic network, which allows for online demonstrations of databases and student interaction at the terminals. The first two-hour session began with a pretest. Appendix B was the pretest used to assess the students' knowledge of information skills. Unaware of students' knowledge of library information-seeking strategies, the librarians sought to determine the students' level of understanding through a pretest. Questions covered the basics of library use such as locating textbooks and journals in the Biomedical Library, when to use the online catalog, when to use MEDLINE, and the use of medical terminology and Boolean logic to define an information need. All of the PBL students did quite well on the pretest. Yet, this was an excellent opportunity to reinforce and advance information-seeking skills which are central educational aims of PBL's problem-solving and life-long learning objectives.[20]

A four-hour sequence of library instruction included an introductory lecture discussing the organization of the biomedical literature and the components of search strategy; it also included an online demonstration of the MELVYL CATALOG. After the review of MELVYL, the session ended with the videotape, "Searching the Medical Journal Literature."[21] The second two-hour session concentrated on the use of MELVYL MEDLINE. Time was devoted to explaining Boolean logic, MeSH, and advanced searching techniques.

Following the library instruction, the four clinical problems were

---

*Trademark of the Regents of the University of California.
**Trademark of the National Library of Medicine.

presented in three two-hour discussion periods in one of the student lecture halls. Librarians attended each of these presentations to assist with suggesting appropriate library resources to use in solving information needs as they arose in the case discussions as well as to guide the students in the use of the library subsequent to each of the presentations.

During the first session of each clinical problem, one fourth-year student portrayed each of the patients while the remaining fourth-year students served as facilitators. The patients told the second-year students, who as a group acted as the examining physician, why he/she was seeking medical attention. Having no prior knowledge of the cases, the second-year students questioned the patients to obtain a full medical history, i.e., chief complaint, history of present illness, medications, allergies, social history, family history, and the review of systems. The facilitator guided the second-year students by introducing questions which required the students to integrate their knowledge of the basic sciences and apply that knowledge to determine the possible differential diagnoses of each of the patients. Neither the patients nor the facilitator offered any pertinent information to the second-year students unless requested. At the end of the first session, the facilitator highlighted a number of open-ended questions left to be resolved by the students. These questions, referred to as "learning issues," were topics which needed clarification to arrive at the proper diagnosis.

During the second session of each clinical problem, the second-year students reported their research from library resources on the learning issues. The students then narrowed their list of possible differential diagnoses by comparing their literature findings with the history and physical examination results of each of the cases. At the end of the second session, the students were assigned additional learning issues to be researched to further reach the concluding diagnosis, while the third session was devoted to discussion of the actual diagnosis and management of the clinical entity.

OBSERVATIONS

The four cases involved neurologic, infectious, cardiac, and neoplastic diseases. During the first presentation of the research on neurologic diseases, the students heavily cited the use of *Harrison's Principles of Internal Medicine* and other similar general medical textbooks.[22] It was interesting to note that the senior students recommended the use of general medical texts. It was evident that they had limited knowledge of information resources. With the librarians present at each session, chances arose for the librarians to intervene with alternative suggestions for finding literature. It was at this stage that specialty textbooks were noted and copies of the current Brandon list, which includes core texts in each discipline, were distributed.[23] Thereafter, the students were assisted on a one-to-one basis with the skills taught in the general library instruction, utilizing the online catalog and MEDLINE to locate books and journal articles appropriate to their cases.

The lack of sophisticated knowledge of the literature on the part of the senior medical students was especially highlighted in the first case, where the diagnoses included "Alzheimer's Disease" and whether this could be definitively diagnosed. The senior students indicated that Alzheimer's could only be diagnosed by a process of exclusion or by autopsy. However, current journal literature cites success with magnetic resonance imaging (MRI) in diagnosing this and other difficult neurologic problems. To highlight this gap, the librarians provided the second-year students with current articles correlating the use of MRI with the diagnosis of Alzheimer's Disease. Fortunately, the senior students were cognizant of their limited literature skills and welcomed the librarians' assistance. Furthermore, they requested that similar instruction be provided for their level.

In another example, one of the second-year students subscribed to *American Family Physician* and recently received a current issue which included an article on one of the diseases he was to research. In a discussion of current therapies, the journal article cited a number of drugs currently in use. Current textbooks, however, noted that the drugs were experimental. By the end of the four cases, the second-year students were made acutely aware of the necessity for consulting the journal literature and not relying on general or specific textbooks. The librarians' role in the students' instruction was evident when it became clear that keeping up with the literature and developing a pattern of life-long learning depended on knowledge of access to current resources.

PROGRAM EVALUATION

With the results of the pretest, the librarians expected the second-year students easily to apply their knowledge to the case assignments. However, even with the addition of the general library instruction, the students were unable to function independently. In light of these experiences, with the pretest not actually testing applicability of knowledge, the posttest for the course, which was modeled in concept after the pretest, no longer proved appropriate and the evaluation mechanism was revised.

Students were asked to evaluate the librarians as instructors, the course content, and course presentation methods of the initial four hours of the formal library component. Additionally, students were asked to comment on the value of the librarian assistance in the problem-based learning cases, as well as to provide comments on additional information they would have found useful. Lastly, in essay form, the students were asked to describe the knowledge they gained as a result of the Biomedical Library's staff interaction for the pilot program in which they were involved.

All 15 participating students returned favorable evaluations. Despite the small number of participants, the information gained can be extrapolated, in that students' comments demonstrated learning had taken place when attached to relevant needs. The librarians will soon have an opportunity to expand this program in the mainstream of the coming academic year with much larger groups of first and second-year students utilizing the same principles. Two suggestions for improvements included allotting more time to the initial presentations and providing one concise list of system commands instead of the large number of handouts used.

As for the knowledge gained, some representative comments follow:

> I greatly increased my knowledge in how to narrow my search results when using MELVYL and MEDLINE and I also became aware of the existence of specialty textbooks and other sources available.

Information skills are absolutely necessary for the medical student and future physician. This course should immediately be implemented in all four years of medical school classes.

The most important thing I learned was knowing how important library work is in medical school, especially in clinical areas.

Before this program, I did not know how to use the journal literature, now I can quickly find pertinent clinical data that is right up-to-date. I also learned when to use books and when journals would be a better source of information.

I learned how medical literature is organized and how to find what I need more easily than I understood before. This information would be beneficial to the entire class during the regular academic year.

CONCLUSIONS

From this preliminary experience, the Biomedical Library staff have drawn several conclusions. First, there is a need for more extensive involvement between the librarians and the faculty in designing the curriculum to incorporate a broader range of resources. The librarians were only involved after the cases had been prepared to assist with guiding the students through the literature. If the cases had required the need for more recently published information along with background information, the journal literature would have been utilized in combination with textbooks, and skills in retrieving journal articles would have been enhanced. Second, attendance by the four librarians at six hours of class presentations each week for four weeks highlighted the labor-intensiveness and the difficulty in maintaining the staffing at the reference desk during this period. It would be helpful to recruit and train staff from other areas to assist with the information management education as well as staff the reference desk. Third, the heavy use of current textbooks necessitates that they be located in a reserve or non-circulating section of the library. Unfortunately, the students found that some of the most current textbooks were checked out from the open stacks, requiring the use of two- to three-year-old editions of some key texts. Finally, the most important conclusion was the demonstration to the students of the benefit of the promotion of active, independent learning, rather than passive learning through the use of the literature within the requirements of their educational process. Formal library instruction was not in itself sufficient to provide the information skills for their needs. Integration of information-seeking skills into the curriculum in a directed sequence of assignments reinforced the applicability of these skills. As the librarians worked with the students on a continued basis with each case, the skills became more meaningful, and less assistance was necessary by the fourth case. If information skills are incorporated at "teachable moments" in the four years of medical school, especially where problem-based learning is utilized, medical students will become sophisticated in managing their information needs and will be prepared to keep abreast of continuing changes in the growth of medical literature. This will allow a higher quality of patient care and research and will facilitate a pattern of life-long learning which will be perpetuated as they become the educators of future generations of medical students.

AUTHOR'S NOTE:

The success of this pilot project coupled with the AAMC publication *Educating Medical Students* have resulted in the full-scale integration of information management skills in the four years of the University of California, Irvine College of Medicine medical school curriculum.

ACME-TRI Report: Educating Medical Students: Assessing Change in Medical Education; the Road to Implementation. Washington, DC, AAMC, 1992.

APPENDIX A

A SAMPLE CASE PRESENTATION

Chief Complaint:	30-yr.-old single white male for routine physical examination as a requirement for employment
History of Present Illness:	Upon questioning has had night sweats once in a while, low grade fever (tactile), weight loss of 10 lbs. in past year—though not trying to lose weight, has a healthy appetite. Swollen glands (neck) for past 6 mos., especially on left side.
Past Medical History	Had bronchitis 4 mos. ago, still has dry cough; had diarrhea off and on for 2 yrs. in Guatemala—says he was told it was giardia—received a shot but had no idea what it was. Received shots before going to Guatemala but didn't know what they were for. No surgeries Asthma Broken arm at 10 yrs. from fall out of tree
Medications:	Takes aspirin occasionally
Allergies:	No known drug allergies
Social History:	Spent 2 yrs. in Guatemala, has been back in states for 6 mos. Smokes 1/2 pack/day for 10 yrs. = 5 pack years Drinks 2 beers/night for 10 yrs. Eats basic meat and potatoes diet Sexually active—encounters with prostitutes in Guatemala with no protection Smoked marijuana
Family History:	Mother & father, sister healthy Heart disease on father's side
Review of Systems:	10 lbs. weight loss over one year Nose slightly red Enlarged mass on left side of neck Liver slightly enlarged

Possible Differential Diagnoses:	HIV	Lipoma
	STD	Sarcoma
	Lymphoma (Hodgkin's)	Tuberculosis
	Oropharyngeal neoplasm	Hepatitis
	Epstein-Barr virus	Lung cancer
	Malaria	
Diagnosis:	Lymphoma (Hodgkin's)	

APPENDIX B

INTRODUCTION TO THE HEALTH SCIENCES LITERATURE

PRETEST

1. *Applied biochemistry of clinical disorders* / edited by Allan G. Gornall ; with 29 contributors. 2nd ed. Philadelphia : Lippincott, c1986.

UCD	HealthSci	QY	90	A63	1986
UCI	Biomed	QY	90	A652	1986
UCI	MedCtr	QY	90	A652	1986
UCLA	Biomed	QY	90	A652	1986

   Given the information for the above reference, how would you find this book in the Biomedical Library?

   _____

   _____

2. Lucarelli, G, Galimberti, M, Polchi, P, Angelucci, E, Baronciani, D.

   Bone marrow transplantation in patients with thalassemia.
   New England Journal of Medicine, 1990 Feb 15, 322(7):417-421.
   Unique ID: 90136741.
   Abstract available; type D 5 SHORT ABS.

   Given the information for the above reference, how would you find this journal article in the Biomedical Library?

   _____

   _____

3. If you know nothing about Down's Syndrome, which source would you consult first:

   a. an encyclopedia of syndromes
   b. a general dictionary
   c. a journal article

Portions of this pretest were extracted from sample questions used by Bradigan and Malarski.[24]

APPENDIX B (continued)

4. The MELVYL^R MEDLINE^R database contains:

   a. references in articles in health sciences journals.
   b. references to health sciences books.
   c. both of the above.

5. The MELVYL^R CATALOG contains:

   a. campus locations of books and journals for only the UCI libraries.
   b. references to journal articles in the field of medicine.
   c. campus locations of books and journals in the UC system.

6. To find a journal article in the field of medicine that has appeared in the literature in the past 6 months, the best database to use is:

   a. MELVYL CATALOG
   b. MELVYL CURRENT CONTENTS
   c. MELVYL MAGS

The next three questions test your ability to pick out the important concepts in a statement of a medical problem. Fill in the blanks with words or phrases you would use to find information on these subjects.

EXAMPLE: I need articles on confidentiality issues and AIDS.

   KEY CONCEPTS WOULD BE: Acquired immunodeficiency syndrome
                          Confidentiality

7. Pregnancy complications resulting from the use of lithium or dilantin.

   KEY CONCEPTS: ──────────────────────────────────

   ──────────────────────────────────

8. Genetic counseling for a patient whose father has Huntington's disease.

   KEY CONCEPTS: ──────────────────────────────────

   ──────────────────────────────────

9. Prognosis of brain carcinoma.

   KEY CONCEPTS: ──────────────────────────────────

   ──────────────────────────────────

10. Searching for information on brain carcinoma, what medical terminology would give you the most complete results:

    a. brain cancer
    b. brain neoplasms
    c. brain tumors

For the most specific results, you will need to combine concepts of a topic you are searching. There are three ways to combine topics. They are using AND, OR, AND NOT. Fill in the blanks with one of the three "combining terms" below:

AND   OR   AND NOT

11. Articles on smoking as a cause of lung cancer.

    Which one of the three combining terms would you use?

    SMOKING _____ LUNG CANCER

12. You are searching for information on nutritional analysis of food, but not animal feed.

    Which one of the three combining terms would you use?

    NUTRITIONAL ANALYSIS _____ ANIMAL FEED

13. You need information on the diagnosis of three hearing disorders: Otitis Media, Otosclerosis, Cholesteatoma.

    Which one of the three combining terms would you use?

    OTITIS MEDIA _____ OTOSCLEROSIS _____ CHOLESTEATOMA

REFERENCES

1. Association of American Medical Colleges. "Physicians for the Twenty-First Century. Report of the Project Panel on the General Professional Education of the Physician and College Preparation for Medicine." *Journal of Medical Education* 59 (Part 2, November 1984):1-208.

2. *Medical Education in the Information Age: Proceedings of the Symposium on Medical Informatics.* Washington, DC: The Association, 1986.

3. Braude, R.M. "Role of Libraries in Medical Education." *Bulletin of the New York Academy of Medicine* 65 (July-August, 1989):728-738.

4. Allegri, F. "Course Integrated Instruction: Metamorphosis for the Twenty-First Century." *Medical Reference Services Quarterly* 4 (Winter 1985):47-66.

5. Dorsch, J.L.; Frasca, M.A.; Wilson, M.L.; and Tomsic, M.L. "A Multidisciplinary Approach to Information and Critical Appraisal Instruction." *Bulletin of the Medical Library Association* 78 (January 1990):38-44.

6. Frasca, M.A.; Dorsch, J.L.; Aldag, J.C.; and Christiansen, R.G. "A Multidisciplinary Approach to Information Management and Critical Appraisal Instruction: A Controlled Study." *Bulletin of the Medical Library Association* 80 (January 1992):23-28.

7. Kimmel, S. "Teaching Third-Year Medical Students to Search MEDLINE." *Medical Reference Services Quarterly* 8 (Fall 1989):69-76.

8. Graves, K.J., and Selig, S.A. "Library Instruction for Medical Students." *Bulletin of the Medical Library Association* 74 (April 1986):126-130.

9. Markert, R.J. "Medical Student, Resident, and Faculty Use of a Computerized Literature Searching System." *Bulletin of the Medical Library Association* 77 (April 1989):133-138.

10. Port, J., and Meiss, H.R. "Teaching Library Skills in Third-Year Clerkships." *Journal of Medical Education* 57 (July 1982):564-566.

11. Simon, F.D. "A Comparison of Two Computer Programs for Searching the Medical Literature." *Journal of Medical Education* 63 (April 1988):331-333.

12. Sarkis, J., and Hamburger, S. "The Impact of the Clinical Librarian." *Journal of Medical Education* 56 (October 1981): 860-862.

13. Proud, V.K.; Schmidt, F.J.; Johnson, E.D.; and Mitchell, J.A. "Teaching Human Genetics in Biochemistry by Computer Literature Searching." *American Journal of Human Genetics* 44 (April 1989):597-604.

14. Burrows, S.; Ginn, D.S.; Love, N.; and Williams, T.L. "A Strategy for Curriculum Integration of Information Skills Instruction." *Bulletin of the Medical Library Association* 77 (July 1989):245-251.

15. Mueller, M.H., and Foreman, G. "Library Instruction for Medical Students during a Curriculum Elective." *Bulletin of the Medical Library Association* 75 (July 1987):253-256.

16. Ben-Shir, R. "Library Instruction Integrated with Patient Management." *Bulletin of the Medical Library Association* 72 (July 1984):310-311.

17. Reidelbach, M.A.; Willis, D.B.; Konecky, J.L.; Rasmussen, R.J.; and Stark, J. "An Introduction to Independent Learning Skills for Incoming Medical Students." *Bulletin of the Medical Library Association* 76 (April 1988):159-163.

18. Leist, J.C., and Kristofco, R.E. "The Changing Paradigm for Continuing Medical Education: Impact of Information on the Teachable Moment." *Bulletin of the Medical Library Association* 78 (April 1990):173-179.

19. Barrows, H.S. *How to Design a Problem-Based Curriculum for the Preclinical Years.* New York: Springer, 1985.

20. Rankin, J.A. "Problem-Based Medical Education: Effect on Library Use." *Bulletin of the Medical Library Association* 80 (January 1992):36-43.

21. Byrd, G. *Searching the Medical Journal Literature.* Kansas City, MO: University of Missouri-Kansas City, School of Medicine, 1980 [videorecording].

22. *Harrison's Principles of Internal Medicine.* 12th ed. New York: McGraw-Hill, 1991.

23. Brandon, A.L., and Hill, D.R. "Selected List of Books and Journals for the Small Medical Library." *Bulletin of the Medical Library Association* 79 (April 1991):195-222.

24. Bradigan, P.S., and Mularski, C.A. "End-user Searching in a Medical School Curriculum: An Evaluated Modular Approach." *Bulletin of the Medical Library Association* 77 (October 1989):348-356.

Chapter 8

Making Housecalls:
An Alternative
to Library Classroom Instruction

Jonquil D. Feldman
Julia K. Kochi

BACKGROUND

In order to keep up with the ever-changing nature of information, libraries continually introduce new services to enhance access. It remains the library's responsibility to ensure that users receive adequate instructional support so that new technology eases access instead of impeding it. To offer a proactive solution to the potential problems of new technology, the Claude Moore Health Sciences Library (CMHSL) at the University of Virginia has developed several different Information Management Educational (IME) programs including scheduled classes, open demonstrations, and individual consultations by appointment.

Like many health sciences libraries, the clientele which CMHSL serves varies from physicians, nurses, and students to secretaries and research assistants. Although every effort is made to offer classes and appointments at convenient times, it is impossible to devise a schedule that suits everyone's needs. Some clients are unable to leave their offices or hospital units due to inadequate coverage; others work a schedule that does not allow them to attend

This chapter was first published in *Medical Reference Services Quarterly*, Vol. 13(2), Summer 1994.

the library's classes. Many sign up for a class and then encounter scheduling conflicts. Some are geographically removed from the main portion of the Health Sciences Center (HSC).

DEVELOPING A NEW SERVICE PROGRAM

To provide an alternative to classes or in-house consultations, the library developed a program called Housecalls, in which librarians provide information management skills to the HSC faculty and staff in a setting outside of the library. The Housecall is designed to incorporate the same type of instruction about information gathering or management offered through the classes and consultations at the library but does so in an office or departmental setting. A Housecall provides personalized service, since the content may be altered to meet the needs of the audience. Some of the services which have been offered in the past include demonstrations of LIS, the library's online catalog; instruction on using PlusNet (produced by CD Plus Technologies), the library's internal online system for searching MEDLINE, CINAHL, or HEALTH; demonstrations of Grateful MED and BRS Colleague; and discussions of bibliographic management software and reprint file management.

In order to offer a personalized service such as Housecalls, which has the potential of being extremely time and labor intensive, the library initially began offering the service to departments rather than individuals. Working under the assumption that most departments hold regularly scheduled meetings, the librarians believed an effective method of reaching users would be to provide instruction at such meetings, some of which have mandatory attendance.

Identifying an Audience

Four types of meetings were initially identified: divisional grand rounds, regular departmental meetings, journal clubs, and specially scheduled meetings. An initial mailing was sent out to a targeted group of divisional chairpersons, laboratory and hospital service directors, and others responsible for coordinating staff meetings. Library instruction was offered as an agenda item for the meetings. The program was also publicized in the library newsletter, which is widely distributed throughout the HSC. Library staff also spoke directly to established contacts in the HSC.

In the three years since this program began, the Information Services staff has done Housecalls at two grand rounds, several departmental meetings where the audience numbered between 30 to 50 people, and numerous small group sessions. Locations have ranged from a nurses' station on the hospital's fourth floor to the Physical Therapy Department of an affiliated hospital located six miles from the HSC. For the Housecall offered to the Respiratory Care Department, CE credit was obtained, and the session was videotaped so others in the department who were unable to attend could later view it.

Developing a Clientele

The response from the initial participants has been sufficient to establish a base of contacts. Meeting coordinators appreciate the convenience of having the instruction in their own meeting rooms and having the content tailored to their needs. Housecalls are now regularly offered as part of the orientation for incoming housestaff. The Consultation Services Coordinator works in conjunction with the Chief Residents of the Internal Medicine, Pediatrics, Surgery, and Dentistry departments to arrange these sessions. The program has expanded beyond physicians and department administrators, and the library staff now works with the coordinators of continuing education programs for the Division of Nursing and allied health professionals. Often a forgotten part of an institution, the nursing and allied health staff are enthusiastic about taking advantage of this service.

Many of the group Housecalls are self-perpetuating now that the initial contact has been made. A large share of new Housecalls has resulted because administrators are becoming more aware of the necessity to access and manage information and want their staff to be competent in these areas. One administrator has invited library staff back for additional sessions. The introduction of the full MEDLINE database in July 1992 increased awareness of the library's systems and made it possible to personally run searches that originally had to be done by the Information Services staff. Clients who previously had little interest in searching are now finding that they need instruction on how to search and how to manage information they retrieve.

Housecalls to Individuals

Realizing that there is a need for assistance with specific problems and that all clients cannot be served through group Housecalls, the library began to offer Housecalls to individuals in September 1991. Information Services staff visit clients in their offices because it makes sense to handle an information problem in a familiar computer environment where the client can best learn how to resolve the problem. Clients benefit from having library staff present while they work through the procedures for connecting to library systems from their own workstations. This is especially important since each workstation is configured differently, and the means of accessing library systems vary widely. Assistance is also offered with specific functions in bibliographic management software. The advantages to clients are in the time saved; the convenience of having a library staff member come to their office and offer an individualized instruction plan; and reduced blood, sweat, and tears.

CONTRASTS BETWEEN HOUSECALLS AND CLASSES

The Housecalls program was developed to complement the scheduled classes offered by the library. Although most group Housecalls are formatted like the classes, the staff time required to prepare for Housecalls tends to be greater. Much like the special classes held in the library, extra preparation time is necessary to formulate good teaching examples tailored to the audience's area of specialty.

Given the uncertain nature of hardware and connections, Housecalls maintain a "fly by the seat of your pants" atmosphere. Up until the final successful connection has been made and the audience is filing out the door, the question remains whether or not the

Housecall will conclude without a hitch. The computer classroom in the library, by contrast, is set up with high-end computers (both IBM compatibles and Macintoshes) and reliable network connections maintained by the Learning Resources Center staff. Although mishaps are not unheard of in the computer classroom, the environment is considerably more controlled, and technical support is available just outside the door.

Negotiation is always involved when scheduling a Housecall. An agreement must be made on a time that best suits the client's calendar as well as ensuring staff coverage in the Information Services Department. Housecalls are sometimes canceled or rescheduled by the requester, often with very little notice; therefore, a certain degree of flexibility on the part of the library staff is necessary. Maintaining a Housecalls program requires aggressive marketing of the service and establishing contacts within the institution. Classes, on the other hand, are regularly scheduled by the library: some are held twice a month, others are offered once a month. Class times are posted in institutional publications and advertised with flyers, and attendees have a variety of times from which to choose.

CONTRAINDICATIONS FOR HOUSECALLS

As convenient as Housecalls may be for the clients, there are circumstances when a Housecall may not be the best solution. A frequent situation occurs when the client wants a library system demonstrated but lacks network or telephone connections. Although the library has developed some "canned" demonstrations for use as backups, they often do not adequately show the functions of the system in which the client is interested. This is especially true in the case of PlusNet. Demonstrating the system without a "live" connection does not show it to its best advantage and gives the incorrect impression that the system is not very versatile or powerful. In these cases, it is recommended that a special class be scheduled in the computer classroom. When the situation is explained, an alternative arrangement can usually be made.

Another situation in which a Housecall may not be appropriate is when the size or location of the meeting room is not conducive to teaching. This has occurred several times in the library staff's experiences. In one instance, the group was too large to crowd around a computer screen, and the room where the Housecall was being offered was too small to set up a projection screen. This is sometimes the case when demonstrations are held in offices. In another instance, the Housecall was held in the Coronary Care Unit where the nurses were constantly interrupted with patient care questions and were distracted by concerns about patients in nearby rooms. The librarian found the interruptions disruptive, and the clients spent more time out of the room than in it. In such cases, it is advisable to reschedule the Housecall as a class in the library or as a series of in-house consultations.

LESSONS LEARNED

The most important lesson learned during the past years can perhaps best be summed up in one word: backups. The importance of having a backup program cannot be emphasized enough. Regardless of the number of times the connections have been checked, the possibility always remains of either the connections failing or the system at the library failing. Because scheduling a Housecall requires so much negotiation, rescheduling the session is usually not a viable option. To lessen the impact of a connection or system failure, demonstrations of LIS and PlusNet have been developed using a software program called SHOW (developed by the Learning Resources Division of the Biomedical Library at the University of California at Los Angeles). SHOW allows the library staff to create an ASCII reproduction of a screen-by-screen display of the system. However, due to the limitations of the SHOW program, it is time-consuming to re-create a complex image. Therefore, the demonstrations contain only the very basics of the systems being shown. Currently, the library is looking into alternative presentation programs that will allow easier re-creation of computer screens. Even though a "canned" presentation is not the optimum method of demonstrating a system, as mentioned earlier, one can at least offer a simple demonstration, which acts as a springboard for further discussion and questions. If necessary, a follow-up session can be scheduled.

Having the proper equipment and accessories is also important. If an online demonstration is part of the session, it is preferable to schedule at least one pre-meeting visit to the room where the Housecall is being presented. However, this cannot always be arranged, and the library staff often has to rely on the word of the department staff. Unfortunately, the level of computer literacy varies greatly from person to person, and it is difficult to gauge the reliability of the information concerning computer hardware and connections. Because of the uncertainty of the type of hardware that will be available, portable equipment from the library is often brought on the trip. The portable equipment includes a laptop or notebook computer installed with a modem and telecommunications software or a network adapter, an LCD pad, and an overhead projector, which are all mounted on a portable cart. The library staff also carries accessories such as a 50-foot phone extension cord in case a connection has to be run in from another office because the phone line in the room is not activated, or the line is digital rather than analog. The latter problem is becoming a more frequent occurrence as digital phone lines are commonly installed in newer buildings. An electrical extension cord and plug adapter are also taken, and the battery for the computer is fully charged to guard against the possibility that an electrical outlet is not available.

CONCLUSIONS

Overall, the Housecalls program has been an educational experience for both staff and clients. From the library's point of view, it offers the staff the opportunity to experience the challenges of an outreach program, such as uncertain teaching environments, with the benefit of being relatively close to the library for technical support. Clients have found the personalized service of Housecalls to be a much appreciated alternative to classes held in the library. Two keys to a successful program are to cultivate contacts within the institution and to aggressively market the program's services. A large amount of flexibility and a certain amount of ingenuity also are invaluable.

Chapter 9

Bibliographic Instruction
in the Hospital Library

Beverly A. Gresehover

The Union Memorial Hospital (UMH), located in Baltimore, Maryland, is a 350-bed patient care, teaching, and research facility specializing in hand surgery, orthopedics, and sports medicine. The Library and Information Resources Division of UMH (UMH Library) serves all affiliated personnel including attending staff, nurses, 130 housestaff and fellows, and over 600 nursing school students in three nursing school programs. The UMH Library is fortunate to have a staff of five–three full-time librarians with MLS degrees, and two Library Assistants with Bachelor's degrees.

The UMH Library provides formalized bibliographic instruction to its clientele in several programs that will be described in this chapter. The bibliographic instruction programs are:

1. Nursing Student Orientations
2. Housestaff Orientations
3. Library Research Techniques Instruction
4. Grateful MED /CD Plus MEDLINE Instruction

NURSING STUDENT ORIENTATIONS

UMH offers nursing students three programs: a one-year Licensed Practical Nurse (LPN) degree program, a three-year Regis-

This chapter was first published in *Medical Reference Services Quarterly*, Vol. 13(3), Fall 1994.

tered Nurse (RN) Diploma program, and a four-year Registered Nurse (RN) Bachelor's Degree program in association with Villa Julie College. Each semester, students in the first and second levels of each nursing program are given a one-hour orientation to the UMH Library which includes an in-depth tour, an introduction to the indexing tools with emphasis on *The Cumulative Index to Nursing and Allied Health Literature* (CINAHL), and an explanation of the nature of nursing literature. Students are taught, many for the first time in their college careers, how to use the card catalog to locate books and audiovisuals, how to find journals on the shelf, and how to locate a journal article on a particular topic using the library's indexes. The National Library of Medicine (NLM) classification system is used in this library.

Later in the semester, nursing instructors assign these students research that involves locating journal articles about a disease or disorder that they have encountered in their clinical work. This gives the students an opportunity to practice the library skills they have learned with the assistance of the library staff. Later in the semester, each student completes an evaluation concerning the value of the library and the library orientation to the student's overall learning experience.

Upper level students are given library instruction which reviews and builds upon the skills they have learned. Research using online bibliographic databases is emphasized.

HOUSESTAFF ORIENTATIONS

Every July, a new group of housestaff–interns, residents, and fellows–begin a year with UMH and are oriented to the UMH Library. The housestaff from each specialty meet with a librarian for an orientation that is geared to their particular patient care and research needs. Each orientation consists of an in-depth tour of the library during which resources of particular interest to that specialty are emphasized. In addition, a brief explanation of the library's indexing tools, online databases, and overall services are explained.

In the past, access to Grateful MED, NLM's user-friendly software for database searching was emphasized and housestaff were encouraged to return to the library for an orientation to this software. Currently, housestaff are introduced to both Grateful MED software and CD Plus MEDLINE searching on CD-ROM.

LIBRARY RESEARCH TECHNIQUES INSTRUCTION

In January 1993, a formal research program was incorporated into the Department of Medicine's Internal Medicine training program to facilitate residents' involvement with research and scholarly activities. As stated in the *Resident Research Manual* (Department of Medicine, The Union Memorial Hospital, December 1992), the fourth goal of the program is to "improve skills with data retrieval from the medical literature via the library and computerized databases."

The UMH Library and the Internal Medicine Division have collaborated to develop a program that introduces medical housestaff to library research techniques through formal lecture and independent research. Residents are given an introduction to library research techniques by a librarian in a formal lecture setting of one or two one-hour sessions, as needed. Discussion topics include:

• organizing an information search,
• using library finding tools,
• using computerized bibliographic databases,
• using Medical Subject Headings (MeSH), and
• practice exercises to reinforce the material presented.

Using overhead transparencies, the librarian presents the use of MeSH in some detail. Boolean search logic, the hierarchical tree structures by which subject headings are organized, and narrowing search retrieval by limiting to the main point of the article or limiting to review articles are some of the concepts discussed.

Residents in the Internal Medicine Division are then assigned an independent research project to be completed during their elective periods. At the beginning of the elective period, each resident meets with a librarian to begin individual instruction in use of the library and its databases. The library staff assists residents with their research projects during the elective period. The resident is responsible for this aspect of the program and the amount of assistance the individual receives from the library is left to the resident's discretion.

In addition to orienting residents to the most rudimentary aspects of library use, such as the shelf organization of the journal collection (often baffling to foreign medical graduates), the library staff may provide instruction in searching MEDLINE on CD-ROM or Grateful MED.

Assignment of research topics and overseeing the progress of the independent research project is the responsibility of the Assistant Chief of the Intensive Care Unit (ICU). This is a particularly useful collaboration since the UMH librarians attend clinical medical rounds in the ICU as part of their outreach service. This enables the librarian and the Assistant Chief of the ICU to share knowledge of patient care needs as well as trends in the ICU, which may be the source for useful research studies, as well as areas in which housestaff knowledge can benefit from library support. The librarians also attend clinical rounds in the Divisions of Obstetrics and Gynecology, Hand Surgery, and Nursing Services.

The formal lecture on library research techniques given to the housestaff in the Department of Internal Medicine is also adapted for annual presentation to the housestaff in the Department of Surgery.

GRATEFUL MED/CD PLUS MEDLINE INSTRUCTION

To ensure that Grateful MED is used efficiently and effectively, the UMH Library has implemented an instructional session for Grateful MED users. To be given a password for free use of Grateful MED, housestaff and nursing students must complete the Grateful MED software tutorial. Experienced users are required to complete only the tutorial chapters that review new commands and software enhancements. After completing the tutorial, the user must complete a brief instructional session with a library staff member. This session reviews basic commands and takes the user through a MEDLINE search prepared by the library staff that illustrates basic searching concepts. At the end of the session, the librarian will assist with any actual searches the user wants to do.

Once this instructional session has been successfully completed, the requester is assigned a password for two to five free hours of access to Grateful MED. The requester may be given additional free hours of access to Grateful MED upon request.

Use of Grateful MED is free to the end user; the library pays NLM at the student searching rate. This system allows the library to budget a specific amount for Grateful MED searching. By requesting a number of passwords from NLM for searching in two-hour and five-hour increments, the library is able to allocate its budget to a large number of end users. Using passwords allows for fair distribution of the end-user searching budget. Requiring that all users complete the orientation/instruction session ensures that they will have had some exposure to the software before embarking on searching independently, thereby increasing the cost-effectiveness of searching as well as the satisfaction level of the end users.

During their orientations, housestaff and upper level nursing students are introduced to the library's CD Plus system for searching MEDLINE on CD-ROM. Upon request, they are oriented to this menu-driven system and may use it during the day by appointment. Recently, access to the library's MEDLINE on CD-ROM was made available to library users at one station in the library from six p.m. until the following morning at eight a.m., and on weekends and holidays. Nursing students and housestaff have after-hours access to the library via their I.D. badges. It is anticipated that access to MEDLINE on CD-ROM during the day by appointment and during evening and weekend hours may eliminate the need to offer Grateful MED searching in the future.

SUMMARY

The nature of bibliographic instruction in this hospital library continues to evolve. As the library makes easy-to-master, menu-driven tools for online searching available to end users, the demand for this service and the accompanying training increases.

The demand for formal sessions covering research techniques is also increasing. Upon request, the library offered an extended research orientation to the housestaff in Obstetrics and Gynecology in May of 1993. An introduction to the use of CD-ROM was included to highlight its usefulness for citation verification, author searches, and for periodic current awareness searches on a particular topic.

The UMH Library staff strive to offer the most current and comprehensive facilities and services to their users. These include automated access to the library's book, journal, and audiovisual holdings using the Data Trek system; online bibliographic searching by library staff and end users using CD Plus MEDLINE on CD-ROM and Grateful MED software; participation in clinical rounds to provide research support for clinical care; and several types of bibliographic instruction. In addition to the informal teaching of library research techniques that the library staff offers on a daily basis, the Library at Union Memorial Hospital is pleased to be able to provide a formalized and evolving bibliographic instruction program.

PART II
TEACHING END-USER SEARCHING

Chapter 10

Teaching End Users the CD Plus MEDLINE Menu Mode in Thirty Minutes

Nicholas G. Tomaiuolo

INTRODUCTION

Teaching may come naturally to some librarians. Yet those fortunate enough to have this skill may require some direction or a framework of reference concerning the specific subject which they are teaching. This is the case with instructing end users in the basic approaches to the CD Plus system of searching MEDLINE. CD Plus is an innovative company residing in New York City. Its product has been previously reviewed.[1]

After using the CD Plus Professional Workstation model to conduct librarian-mediated MEDLINE searches in the Information Services Department of the Stowe Library at the University of Connecticut Health Center for one year, two CD Plus Patron Workstations were purchased and made available for end users.[2]

The Patron Workstation can be used in either a menu mode, or in a direct searching mode. If the end user chooses to search directly, it is assumed that he will know how to qualify terms, how to correctly enter authors' names, and how to enter other system commands. In the menu mode, much less is left to the end user's memory. Initially, it was believed that users searching in the menu mode would require very little assistance. The menus prompt the user for input. Members of the Information Services staff invariably used the di-

This chapter was first published in *Medical Reference Services Quarterly*, Vol. 10(4), Winter 1991.

rect mode so the eccentricities of the menu mode were not, at first, apparent to them. As they were called upon to provide ad hoc instruction at the two Patron Workstations and looked more closely at the menu mode's features and pitfalls, it became obvious that some instruction would be needed if patrons were to realize many of the powers of the CD Plus system.

CD Plus has depth; there are numerous ways to approach a search question. Additionally, what CD Plus presents on its initial menu screen is only a portion of what the system is capable of doing. (The intent of this chapter is to help colleagues at medical libraries incorporate some of the most direct techniques for imparting information about the power of CD Plus within short time constraints.) CD Plus is a well-constructed, richly embellished access to MEDLINE; it lends itself to quick learning and quick teaching. Users who become proficient in searching the menu mode will view it as a precursor to direct searching.

The menu mode, however, is not without its shortcomings. There is no actual documentation for use with the menu mode; it is presumed that none is necessary because the system prompts the user for all input. The system does not have the capability of using the logical operator "not." Subject headings tagged as minor headings are not readily retrievable. Explodes, treeing, and other finer points of searching are available to the user, but are not made readily apparent. The tutorial that is included with the CD Plus MEDLINE software can be read while online or downloaded for later study. It does not teach that these aforementioned features are available–they can only be revealed by someone who has experimented with the system, has accrued a knowledge of the "tricks," and knows the system well.

WHAT IS NOT TAUGHT

CD Plus has several capabilities that are too time-consuming to teach to end users who will be searching in the menu mode. Instructors should bear in mind that teaching these features would not be "counterproductive." If the objective, however, is to provide a basic overview of the system, instruction should omit the following points: (1) "Treeing"; (2) accessing the permuted index; (3) using the "scope" command to see definitions and indexing notes; (4) "Changing Files" (where this option is available); and (5) pre-exploding subheadings (i.e., therapy); which became available with the January 1991 Global update. Time is a factor in these brief encounters which are meant to get users started. The ability to search the system directly in a command mode should definitely be mentioned. As the instruction proceeds, appropriate comments may be added which will encourage users to access the direct mode when they are more experienced. Although the temptation exists to provide insight into every unique feature of the system, it is wisest to resist and cover only the most basic points initially.

DEMONSTRATING THE BASICS

The instructor should begin by informing users as to the literal-ness of the system. The patron must understand that the helpful messages/hints/directives shown on the screens should be read and followed. When the computer boots the system and the first CD Plus screen comes up, users should be aware that the direction to "x" a choice is literally what must be done. It is always surprising to find the number of users who do not "x" an option but simply, press the enter key successively only to hear responding "beeps" signalling their error. The instruction to "Press any key to con-tinue" means just that: press ANY key.

THE SEARCH OPTION MENU

As soon as the user enters "y" to the question "do you wish to use menus?", the search option menu will appear as a window on the CD Plus screen (see Figure 10.1). The instructor then describes the possible types of searches in consecutive, logical steps.

SUBJECT SEARCHING

Option "a" is subject searching. This is an opportunity to illus-trate several features, most important "majoring" and "mapping."

FIGURE 10.1. Search Option Menu

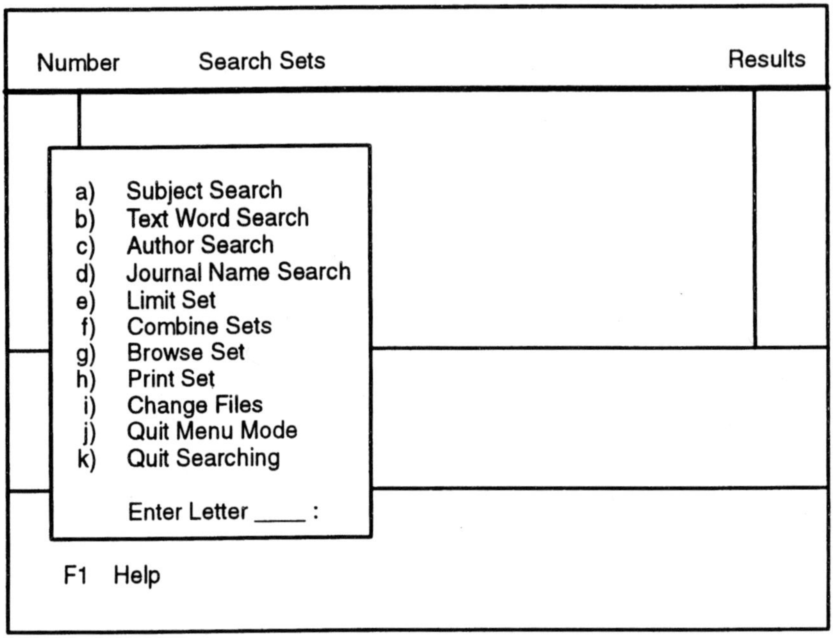

Number	Search Sets	Results

a) Subject Search
b) Text Word Search
c) Author Search
d) Journal Name Search
e) Limit Set
f) Combine Sets
g) Browse Set
h) Print Set
i) Change Files
j) Quit Menu Mode
k) Quit Searching

Enter Letter _____ :

F1   Help

It may also be used as a point of departure to demonstrate the use of the print permuted and annotated *Medical Subject Headings* tools. The instructor should explain that the system is somewhat intelligent; the software has the power to map cross-references to preferred Medical Subject Headings. Two good examples are accomplished by typing either "aids" or "cancer" after entering "a" to select the subject searching option. CD Plus will provide immediate retrieval for MeSH terms entered in correct format. If the entered term is a cross-reference, CD Plus will immediately "map" to the preferred entry. If the entered term is not a Medical Subject Heading but is related to one or more terms from the controlled vocabulary, the user is presented with a list of Medical Subject Headings from which to choose a term to search. If the entered term cannot be matched or does not relate to any Medical Subject Heading, zero results will be retrieved.

As an example, a user needing articles on "enteric fever" might enter these words at the subject search option. CD Plus will immediately inform the user that the preferred entry form is "typhoid." Figure 10.2 shows the format in which mapped headings are retrieved. If the entered term is not only a subject heading itself, but is also a word in one or more other headings, all the possible entries will be offered to the searcher; the searcher must select the single most relevant heading. Therefore, if the user entered "typhoid," the next screen would list "typhoid" as well as "typhoid-paratyphoid vaccines."

Following retrieval of a valid heading, the user will then be presented with a list of topical subheadings which relate to the majored MeSH term. Moving the cursor up or down and selecting (or deselecting) subheadings with an "x" is the next step. Of course, the user has the option of choosing no particular aspect of the subject; this is done by "xing" nothing, but simply hitting the enter key.

It should be noted that retrieval is always of terms as major Medical Subject Headings (unless the term's only postings are as a minor heading) and this is signified by the system preceding the term with an asterisk (*); this bears discussion with the end users. It is imperative to inform users that the only way to be certain of retrieving all the citations indexed to a term, whether it is used as a major or a minor heading, is to enter "a" (select subject searching), type the heading, and complete the entry with a slash (/). Retrieval from terms so entered is shown in Figure 10.3, line two. Although the subject heading must be entered with a slash (/), it will not be shown with a slash (/) upon retrieval. Confirmation that the user has retrieved both major and minor uses of the term is that the subject heading is not preceded by the asterisk (*) when it appears on the monitor. As the instructor makes the end user cognizant of this secret–it is not covered in any of the menu mode's help screens or in the tutorial–the end user should also be told that no subheadings will be offered if the term is so entered. The only means by which to include subheadings at this point is to know what subheadings are available for a particular term and to follow the slash (/) with the proper two-letter abbreviations (see Figure 10.3, line seven). A convenient way of discovering what possible subheadings exist for

FIGURE 10.2. Format in Which Mapped Headings Are Retrieved

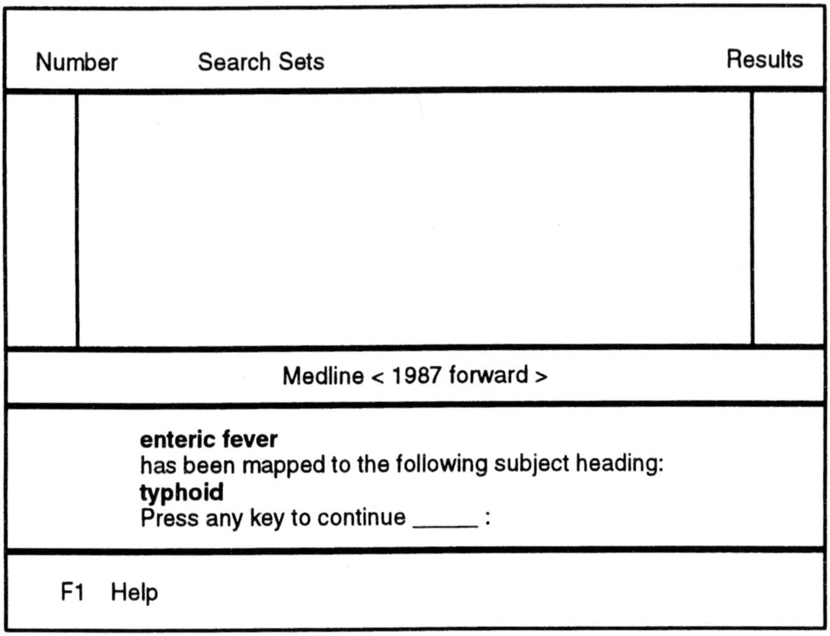

Number	Search Sets	Results

Medline < 1987 forward >

enteric fever
has been mapped to the following subject heading:
typhoid
Press any key to continue _____ :

F1   Help

a given topic is to initially search it as a major heading, and then inspect the list of offered subheadings. The instructor can eliminate discussion of these points, but it is unfair to lead the user to believe retrieval is comprehensive by merely entering a subject heading at the subject search option. The system's default to major headings is probably not an oversight of CD Plus's software developers, but it is not necessarily a great help to searchers, particularly since no alternative is evident to the uninitiated menu user.

TEXT WORD SEARCHING

By entering "b" from the menu option window, the Text Word search capability is accessed. The CD Plus hint on the screen will instruct the user to "enter a word or phrase to be searched in titles or abstracts." CD Plus will allow right-hand-truncation using a "#"

(substitutes for one letter), ":" (substitutes for one or more letters), or "$" (substitutes for one or more letters). The system will also allow internal truncation for one or more letters using any of the same symbols. This is perhaps too detailed a subject to discuss, however, within a short time period.

In the example presently being considered, the user has decided that more specific information concerning typhoid, to which CD Plus mapped the entry of enteric fever as an endemic disease, is required. The instructor types in "endemic disease" and presses the enter key. The instructor should mention that several words may be entered and searched in adjacent order, for example, "late luteal phase dysphoric disorder." CD Plus searches for the words in adjacent order, and then separates retrieval into two sets. One set represents retrieval from the titles while the second set represents retrieval from the abstracts (see Figure 10.3, lines three and four).

This is an opportunity to introduce end users to the "Combine sets" option. The instructor may explain Boolean operators, while noting that to maximize retrieval for the concept of "endemic disease," searchers would logically want to "or" the two sets together (see Figure 10.3, line five). The standard graphic of three Venn diagrams may be used to illustrate the function of the operators. The instructor should tell the end users that CD Plus does not allow the use of "not" in the menu mode.

COMBINING SETS

The next point to cover in the 30-minute instruction session is option "f," "Combine Sets" on the menu. CD Plus prompts with "Enter set number to combine (separate by space)." Experienced searchers will perceive the protocol for combining sets as straightforward; new users may be justifiably confused. Although this format follows no intrinsic logic, it gets the job done. The next prompt asks the user to specify a Boolean operator to combine the sets. CD Plus asks that the users type "o" for "or" or type "a" for "and."

At this juncture, the instructor can recap everything that has transpired while mentioning to the end users that the next logical step in the process is to combine the topic "endemic disease" again, as shown in search step five from Figure 10.3, with the subject of

FIGURE 10.3. System Retrieval

Number	Search Sets	Results
1	*typhoid	445
2	typhoid	524
3	endemic (ti) adj disease (ti)	6
4	endemic (ab) adj disease (ab)	51
5	3 or 4	57
6	5 and 2	2
7	typhoid/ep	78
8	limit 7 to english	52
9	limit 8 to review	5

Medline < 1987 forward >

The last search retrieved 5 citations. They have been put into set number 9. Press any key to continue _____ :

F1 Help

typhoid as retrieved in search step two of the same figure. Attendees can be involved by being asked which operator to use to find citations which will have both criteria in common.

BROWSING

At this point, the search has succeeded in locating citations on typhoid as an endemic disease. The instructor should suggest browsing and select option "g," "Browse Set" from the option window. As the system begins to bring up the first reference, this is a good time to explain the elements of the MEDLINE Unit Record. After detailing the basic information that the citation provides, the instructor can emphasize the usefulness of Medical Subject Headings and subheadings by pointing out that, in the case of this search, epidemiology ("ep") might be the appropriate subheading to include in the next search to expand the retrieval, inasmuch as the citations on typhoid and endemic disease contained that subheading in their records (see Figure 10.4).

REFINING THE SEARCH

The instructor can now unleash the power of CD Plus by going back to the option window, selecting "a," and entering TYPHOID/ ep (see Figure 10.3, line seven). Retrieval is considerably larger. The end users can now be taught the value of the "Limit Set" option "e." The instructor may choose, for example, to limit to English and Review Articles, while being certain to make the participants aware of the other valuable limits: humans, animals, age groups, AIM journals, female subjects, latest update, and so forth (see Figure 10.3, lines eight and nine).

It is important for the instructor to remind users to notice the various function keys and to note their capabilities, one of which is F3, "Print Citation." After depressing F3, the user is presented with a choice of print parameters. The instructor should then note that the fields which are chosen for printing at this point will be the fields to which the system will default for every print command issued during the remainder of the present browsing session. Patrons are often vexed when the printer does not immediately begin working after they have completed the first print command. Again, the literalness of CD Plus must be mentioned: nothing will print until the user is "Finished Browsing" and has pressed F1.

AUTHOR SEARCHING

This search is similar to "neighboring" on Elhill databases, "rooting" on BRS, or "expanding" on DIALOG. From the option window, the user should select "s" and simply enter the author's last name, a space, and first initial. CD Plus immediately transfers the input to a screen which shows the 100 entries that alphabetically

FIGURE 10.4. Citation in MEDLINE Unit Record Format

Citation 1 to 5

Unique Identifier
  90337716
Authors
  Schwartz E.   Shlim DR.
Title
  Enteric fever among Israeli travelers in Nepal: the need for typhoid
  vaccination.
Institution
  CIWEC International Clinic, Kathmandu, Nepal.
Journal
  Israel Journal of Medical Sciences. [JC:gy0] 26(6):325-7, 1990 Jun
Mesh Headings
  adult. *bacterial vaccines/tu [therapeutic use]. female. human.
  incidence. israel. male. nepal. *travel. **typhoid**/ep [epidemiology].
Abstract
  Enteric fever is still an **endemic disease** in many developing countries.

F1 End Browsing	F4 Skip to Citation	n Next Citation
F2 Find Similar Citations	F5 Flag Citation	p Previous Citation
F3 Print Citation		

---

surround and include the user's input. Using the cursor and "x" key, the searcher then selects one or more names; the program will "or" the selections together automatically into one search statement (see Figure 10.5, line one).

JOURNAL TITLE SEARCH

Journal title searching is popular with end users who need to find citations quickly and already have identified journals which may discuss their topic. It is a straightforward matter to enter the correct option from the Search Option Menu "d," "Journal Title Search," and type as many letters from a journal title to make it unique from other possible entries; but, as CD Plus warns, "do not abbreviate."

FIGURE 10.5. Retrieval of Author, Journal Title Searches

Number	Search Sets	Results
1	schneiderman-h (au)	34
2	md computing (jn)	168
3	*national library of medicine (u.s.)	27
4	2 and 3	1

Medline < 1987 forward >

The last search retrieved 1 citation. It has been put into set number 4. Press any key to continue _____ :

F1   Help

The instructor should explain the difference between truncating a journal title and using an abbreviation as given in a bibliography or in the *List of Serials Indexed for Online Users*. If the user is trying to locate articles in *MD Computing*, only "md com" need be entered. As with author searches, the input is immediately entered into a dictionary of alphabetically ordered titles from which the searcher uses the cursor and "x" key to select the desired title(s). At this point, the instructor can look for specific articles in the retrieved journal title by performing another subject search followed by the combine option to "and" the results. Majoring and mapping can also be reinforced here. In the example in Figure 10.5, lines two to four, the searcher typed in the letters "nlm" as a subject; it was mapped to "national library of medicine (u.s.)," and automatically retrieved as a major term. A more clinically illustrative example would be to enter the "journal of the american dental assoc" and then combine it with the Text Word "mouthwashes."

QUESTIONS ANYONE?

The floor may be opened to the attendees. Questions are likely to include "what if my term is not a heading?" That would be an opportunity to stress the use of Text Words. Actual searches may be requested by the attendees and these may be tackled or deferred at the instructor's discretion. Even the best searcher's credibility may be shattered by an online gaffe.[3]

SUMMARY

Guidance through the CD Plus menu mode is warranted and has proved worthwhile. The Stowe Library's Information Services Department offers instruction once per week; the session usually lasts 30 minutes but may run longer if the attendees are particularly astute or enthusiastic. Individuals or classes may also request instruction at times that are better suited to their schedules.

Librarians who search CD Plus on a daily basis will undoubtedly become facile with the direct searching mode. New end users will probably enjoy more success by using the menu mode. The menu mode does not provide documentation; therefore, a modified text of this article including the illustrations might be considered an adequate print manual for the menus. However, many of the system capabilities cannot be used unless they are taught by an experienced operator. Such a basic but necessary introduction requires approximately one-half hour. The pace will be brisk, and time for extraneous experimentation is unlikely. A successful instruction session is a result of preparation rather than improvisation. If the specific interests of the clientele in attendance are known in advance, a reworking of the examples would be appropriate.

Although no formal evaluation of this instruction technique has been made, most attendees express an appreciation and understanding of the system's capabilities by the end of the session. Tangible feedback comes from seeing an end user who has participated in instruction return to the workstation on an ongoing basis to search the database successfully.

NOTES

1. Brahmi, F.A., and Kaneshiro, K. "CD Plus: MEDLINE on CD-ROM." *Medical Reference Services Quarterly* 9 (Spring 1990): 29-41.

2. Formerly the Stowe Library offered another CD-ROM product to the public for MEDLINE searching. CD Plus has proven far superior in its ease of use, its menu set-up, its explanations of various features (e.g., subheadings, print parameters, use of limit options). Patrons express great enthusiasm and satisfaction with the system. Two CD Plus Patron workstations are available at this library and both offer MEDLINE searching back to 1987. This span of years requires two CD-ROM drives per workstation. The Stowe Library's CD Plus Patron Workstations use IBM PS/2 Model 30 hardware with 286 microprocessors and color monitors. The Information Services Department uses an IBM-compatible with a 386 microprocessor. Eight CD-ROM drives provide every year of MEDLINE back to 1966. Included among the features the staff utilize are executing SDIs. Performing searches on the HEALTH database while eliminating overlapping MEDLINE citations with a selection from the limit options is also possible. Contact CD Plus at 333 Seventh Avenue, 6th floor, New York, New York 10001 (telephone: 212-563-3006).

3. Bell, S.J. "Using the Live Demo in *Online* Instruction" *Online* 14 (May 1990):38-42.

Chapter 11

A Graphical Teaching Aid
for Explaining MEDLINE
and Access to It

Dudee Chiang

BACKGROUND

Assisting library users in doing their own computer searching on
MEDLINE has become a common service among health sciences
libraries. Medical librarians have taken on the responsibilities of
teaching and supporting such a service. There is more than one way
to access MEDLINE, and some libraries provide several of them.
For example, the Norris Medical Library at the University of Southern California (USC) has the complete data of the most current ten
years of MEDLINE loaded on the University's mainframe computer; it is one of more than a dozen databases on the USCInfo
system. Before MEDLINE was available on USCInfo, Norris used
to have the most current three years data on compact disc (CD-
ROM) through Compact Cambridge™. As part of the Regional
Medical Library system, Norris also provides instruction to local
health professionals on using the Grateful MED™ software. Until
recently, Norris offered workshops on searching MEDLINE with
the National Library of Medicine's (NLM) command language.

With the diverse ways to access MEDLINE, some patrons confuse MEDLINE with the various ways to reach it. Many users do

This chapter was first published in *Medical Reference Services Quarterly*, Vol.
11(4), Winter 1992.

not understand that the basic information is the same in all "versions" of MEDLINE, only the software for retrieving and displaying the information is different.[1] A faculty member who was trained with MEDLINE on CD-ROM insisted students do their assignment on CD-ROM even though the Library had switched to USCInfo MEDLINE. Students and residents coming from other institutions would ask for MELVYL MEDLINE, miniMEDLINE, or CD-ROM, and be somewhat confused when they were first shown USCInfo MEDLINE. And some researchers wondered about the differences between using Grateful Med or USCInfo MEDLINE, and having their own CD-ROM MEDLINE in their laboratory. Clearly there was a need to develop a teaching aid to help in explaining the relationships between the database MEDLINE and the various ways to access it.

THE MEDLINE DIAGRAM

Figure 11.1 was developed to help patrons visualize that there is more than one way to access MEDLINE. It was hoped that "a picture can tell more than a thousand words." With this diagram, most patrons would understand that there is only one MEDLINE database, but many different routes to reach it. The diagram is composed of several elements, each element representing either a stage in creating the MEDLINE database or a way to access it. The elements are:

(a) Biomedical journal literature: articles published in more than 3,000 biomedical journals are the raw materials for MEDLINE.

(b) The indexing process: all articles are indexed with Medical Subject Headings. Other information related to the content of the article, such as Chemical Abstract Registry number(s) or gene sequences, is also added to the record when it is entered into MEDLINE.

(c) The MEDLINE database at the National Library of Medicine.

(d) Printed products: *Index Medicus* and other printed indices are created from the MEDLINE database.

(e) Access through another mainframe computer: universities (e.g., USC) or commercial vendors (e.g., BRS, DIALOG) lease

MEDLINE data from National Library of Medicine, and load the data on their own mainframe computer. Usually each institution has different software to read and retrieve information from the database.

(f) Direct dial-up: through a modem, a telephone line, and communications software, a user can call up the computer at the National Library of Medicine directly and search MEDLINE using NLM's command language.

(g) Dial-up through local front-end software: Grateful MED™ falls into this category. With front-end software, users do not have to memorize the tedious searching commands. This type of software usually includes a communications module, which also helps to simplify the dialing and logging-on/off procedures.

(h) CD-ROM: CD-ROM publishers lease MEDLINE data from NLM and distribute it on the compact discs. When one searches MEDLINE on a CD-ROM disc, all interactions occur between the user's computer and the CD-ROM player.

(i) User's computer: the computer or terminal a person uses to access and search MEDLINE.

USING THE DIAGRAM

A transparency was made from this diagram for librarians to use in their classes. It has been shown at course-related sessions for medical and pharmacy students, as well as at library-sponsored Information Management Workshops. When the diagram is included in a session, it is usually shown during the introduction. It gives students a framework for where MEDLINE comes from, which route of access the particular session is discussing, and the relative relationships between the systems for those students that have searched MEDLINE on a different system.

Currently, Norris Medical Library offers two separate Information Management Workshops on searching MEDLINE through USCInfo: Basic USCInfo Searching and Advanced MEDLINE Searching. This diagram helps in conveying the idea that there are two types of knowledge and skills involved in doing a computer search: skills to manipulate the computer and knowledge about the database. At the Basic USCInfo Searching workshop, students learn the commands to navigate within USCInfo; these commands are system-specific. At the Advanced MEDLINE Searching workshop, attendees learn general MEDLINE features such as Medical Subject Headings, major focus, subheadings, and MeSH tree structures. These features are unique to MEDLINE; no matter which version of MEDLINE a person is searching, they should be available. This diagram shows that basic knowledge about MEDLINE and MeSH is transferrable. Only the commands for interacting with the computer system may be different.

COMPOSING THE DIAGRAM

The diagram shown in Figure 11.1 was drawn with MacDraw™ on a Macintosh SE™ computer. Most of the figures (a,c,e,f,g,h,i) were assembled from rectangles and circles, with different shadings. The books (b,d) were "cut-and-pasted" from HyperCard™ Art Ideas stacks. With prior knowledge of MacDraw, it took the author approximately five hours to complete this diagram.

The diagram was purposely simplified to make it clear and easy to understand. Depending on definitions, there can be more than four ways to access MEDLINE. For example, BRS, DIALOG, and locally mounted MEDLINE at different institutions can be considered as different routes of access. However, they are grouped together here in (e) as one category. Similarly, there are nearly a dozen CD-ROM publishers making MEDLINE available on CD-ROM; only one disc is shown in (h). This diagram was not meant to be a detailed map of all possible ways of accessing MEDLINE.

Figure 11.1 is the generic version of this diagram, without any printed description. Figure 11.2 is a variation of Figure 11.1 with the appropriate routes for users at USC spelled out. Figure 11.2 can be used by any library; in fact, it can be used to describe other databases with multiple access as well.

CONCLUSION

When used properly, visual images can illustrate relationships among different computer systems clearly and easily. With the pro-

FIGURE 11.1. Generic MEDLINE Diagram

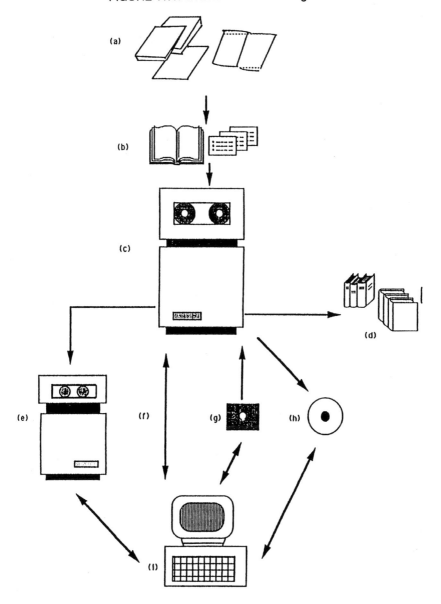

FIGURE 11.2. USC MEDLINE Diagram

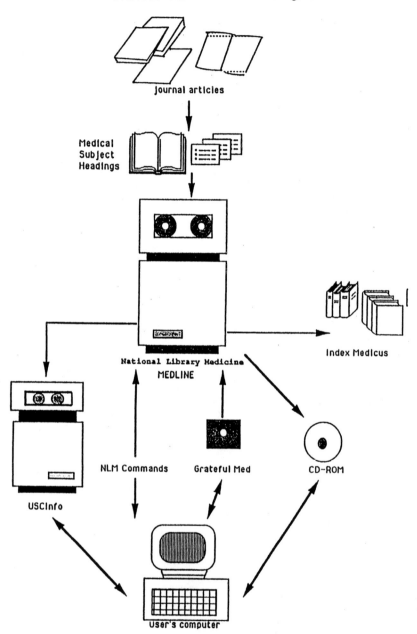

liferation of graphics and desktop publishing software, both on IBM and Apple platforms, it is not difficult to compose such graphics. This diagram is just one example of how graphics software can be used for information management education.

NOTE

1. The coverage may be different among institutions, too. Number of years available varies, and some institutions have only a subset of the entire database.

Chapter 12

Teaching Computer Searching to Health Care Professionals: Why Does It Take So Long?

Julia Sollenberger
Bernie Todd Smith

Medical reference librarians who are teaching or who contemplate teaching a course on computerized database searching must realize the importance of time factors involved in the development of a course. For example, one of these factors is lesson preparation by the instructor. Another factor is the time required by end users to listen and absorb the lessons that identify concepts and provide instruction to search an online database. Search intermediaries know from experience that this type of learning takes a great deal of time. Because search training is demanding, most librarians may be limited by other projects and staff shortages as to what can be offered for end-user search training. The medical literature is replete with descriptions of computer searching courses that range from one hour to 20 hours in length.[1] The librarians at Rochester General Hospital and at the University of Rochester School of Medicine and Dentistry have jointly developed a curriculum[2] for teaching a course ranging from eight to 20 hours, depending on the targeted audience. The basic question one might have concerning this course is, "Why does it take so long?" This chapter examines the course content and the teaching commitment required and addresses the pros and cons of teaching a longer course. Finally, this

This chapter was first published in *Medical Reference Services Quarterly*, Vol. 6(4), Winter 1987.

chapter discusses the advantages to a library of offering any educational program for computer searching, whether it be a long course, a short course, or even a demonstration.

In the Rochester teaching programs, course planning began with the goal of developing and teaching a comprehensive curriculum for those who wish to become sophisticated searchers. Such a goal implies a relatively long course, spanning a minimum of eight hours and designed to include conceptual as well as practical material. The course attendees learn the structure of the MEDLINE database, and they understand the indexing process along with the advantages of searching with a controlled vocabulary. Accordingly, they learn the interrelationship of the *Annotated Medical Subject Headings,* the *Permuted Medical Subject Headings,* and the *Tree Structures.* The course also teaches the use of cross-references, major and minor descriptors, subheadings, and check tags. In addition, attendees learn topic analysis as a preliminary to search strategy formulation. Topic analysis includes defining important concepts, identifying the relationship between the concepts, and then using Boolean operators to enter the strategy online. The course instructors encourage participants to use a search worksheet to help them organize their thoughts and convert those thoughts into an effective search strategy.

In addition to the conceptual skills mentioned above, the course includes a series of online exercises using BRS Colleague. Such practice is deemed essential toward helping students "solidify" the search process. Supervised practice during scheduled class time enables students to execute adequate searches on their own once the course is over and increases the probability of their becoming frequent searchers. One library has reported that the students taking a longer course demonstrate "greater confidence and understanding of online searching gained from successfully completing several required written and hands-on exercise sets."[3]

At the University of Rochester the librarians offer a 20-hour preclinical elective to medical students. Working in pairs at each computer, the medical students complete seven sets of online exercises with four or five questions in each set. The medical students' need for computer searching is not as immediate as that of other health care professionals; the students will not have as much occasion to utilize their own search topics immediately after the course. Because of the time lag between content and application, the course is designed to include more in-class practice for medical students.

In contrast to the medical students, the faculty, staff, and residents who commit the extensive time required to take the course do have their own search topics and a greater sense of immediacy about learning to search. The course participants complete only one or two questions from each set of exercises. The reduced online time allows the librarians to offer the faculty, staff, and residents a condensed, eight-hour version of the course. Although it is less than half as long as the computer searching elective for medical students, this eight-hour course is still relatively long when compared to end-user search training offered by many other institutions. For both the 20-hour or the eight-hour course, the hands-on exercises remain the most time consuming, and yet, the most essential portion of computer search training.

The librarian's time commitment in preparing for and teaching a computer searching course is even more demanding than the time requirements imposed on the students. The collaboration between librarians at the University of Rochester and Rochester General Hospital required approximately 200 professional hours and 100 clerical hours for curriculum development and production.[4] Developing one's own teaching curriculum can be a tremendous effort. Even if a course is taught using a curriculum developed elsewhere, the following list of time-consuming tasks must be completed before the first class:

- Adapt the curriculum to one's own situation and teaching style.
- Schedule and advertise the course.
- Prepare hardware and software configurations.
- Understand the course material thoroughly by trying out many of the examples in advance.
- Devise relevant online demonstrations.
- Prepare lecture notes and additional instructional aids.

After all this preparation, instructors still have to devote much time to the teaching process itself. Experience has shown, however, that an organized teaching effort is optimal; the use of the instructor's time is maximized when questions are anticipated and answered in a group setting, rather than on an individual basis. Unfortunately, group sessions, as opposed to individual help sessions, cannot always occur during regular library hours. It may be necessary to plan for some evening classes to accommodate the busy daytime schedules of residents and other health professionals. A course registration fee should also be considered. Requiring such a fee makes students feel that the course is valuable and encourages consistent class attendance. Finally, planners must consider the number of potential instructors in the library as well as time availability of each instructor before developing training strategies.

Both the librarians and the students participating in an in-depth searching course face significant time requirements if they wish to be successful in their endeavor. The longer course is definitely designed for the committed learner, not for someone who wants merely to see a quick demonstration of computer searching. But even medical students who take the comprehensive course, and subsequently do not search regularly, find that their use of the *MeSH* vocabulary and their ability to analyze search topics are transferable skills. How many library users would sit through a lengthy discussion of cross-references in *MeSH* if it were not under the guise of learning to use a computer?

Before determining the necessary time allocations, instructors must first determine what students want to accomplish in the course. Only then can the library staff define their objectives for teaching. In the two Rochester programs, the students who were demanding such a course indicated that they were frustrated by their inability to perform an efficient search which retrieved the most relevant references. Therefore, the goal of these teaching programs is to train proficient searchers. At other institutions the demands of students might indicate the need for a short, one to two-hour session. A shorter course might provide an overview of computer searching and probably would not include practice with *MeSH* or with online exercises. The librarian's objective in teaching an overview course might be to establish the librarian as an expert in the new technology. A shorter, overview course is also helpful in reaching a larger audience. Furthermore, the library staff can generate significant public relations value from this wide exposure.

Regardless of the length of the course offered, there are important reasons for demonstrating the librarian's familiarity with user-friendly systems and their expertise in the technical field of online bibliographic searching. First of all, librarians can enhance their image if they assume the role of educators and consultants, as well as organizers of information. At the University of Rochester, the librarians gained the credibility of being instructors of a preclinical elective. It may be unfortunate, but many people appear to regard more highly those librarians who demonstrate computer skills in addition to their traditional library skills. Teaching the course can also create new library users. After offering the searching course to attending physicians, the hospital librarians found that the physicians' awareness and use of the library increased. The computer searching course can also make the library more visible in the overall institution. At Rochester General Hospital, the library was mentioned in the annual report of the Quality Assurance Committee as offering training which "gives the user some computer literacy as well as a working knowledge of the resource tools available in our library."[5]

Teaching the course can reap additional benefits. The course places the librarian in the role of instructor, which can serve to enhance collegial relationships between librarians and physicians, especially if an informal, workshop-like atmosphere is established. Teaching can also encourage departmental cooperation. The Computer Services staff at Rochester General Hospital responded to the publicity about the computer searching course by agreeing to develop with the library staff a computer literacy course during 1987. The searching course can also serve as a vehicle for getting computers into the library. The libraries involved in this project have received hardware funding from the medical staff, the Department of Medical Education, the Dean's Office, and various clinical departments. The libraries now have five new computers which are used in teaching computer searchings. But most important, the course serves as excellent advertising for the expertise and specialized skills of the librarians. As a result of the course, more users are now aware of how difficult, complicated, and time-consuming it is to produce quality online searches.

Many librarians have other commitments which do not allow

them to develop a teaching program in computer searching. One good alternative is to demonstrate the use of the system to library clientele. Even a small demonstration provides good public relations for the library and helps to display the librarian's expertise with the user-friendly systems.

Each librarian who contemplates training end users to search for themselves must decide among several alternatives. These include offering a comprehensive course, a short overview, or brief demonstrations. In fact, the ideal situation is likely to involve all three types of programs at different times to meet the needs of a wide range of library users. Whatever teaching program is developed, librarians involved in end-user training will reap the long-term benefits from their efforts. The role that librarians assume in demystifying various online systems sets the stage for further involvement in the acquisition and development of larger, locally integrated online information systems.

NOTES

1. An example of the literature discussing short courses is Slingluff, D., Lew, Y., and Elsan, A. "An End-User Search Service in an Academic Health Sciences Library." *Medical Reference Services Quarterly* 4 (Spring 1986):11-21.

2. The authors and their colleagues use a curriculum developed by the authors and Kathryn Nesbit, Reference/Interlibrary Loan Librarian, Edward G. Miner Library, University of Rochester School of Medicine and Dentistry. Copies of the text are available from the authors.

3. Linder, Gloria A.; Lenon, Richard A.; Su, Valerie; Wible, Joseph G.; and Stangl, Peter. "Training the End User: The Stanford University Medical Center Experience." In: Wood, M. Sandra, Horak, Ellen Brassil, and Snow, Bonnie, eds. *End User Searching in the Health Sciences.* New York: The Haworth Press, 1986, p. 123.

4. The costs of developing the curriculum were subsidized, in part, by a grant from the New York State Hospital Library Program. This grant was administered by the Rochester Regional Library Council.

5. *Annual Report of the Quality Assurance Committee.* Rochester, NY: Rochester General Hospital, 1985.

Chapter 13

End-User Training:
Does It Make a Difference?

Joanne G. Marshall

Remote online databases such as MEDLINE, EMBASE, and BIOSIS have been accessible for many years through search intermediaries located in libraries and information centers. Such databases provide health professionals with interactive access to the latest published information on research and patient care topics. Vendors of online and the newer CD-ROM products are attempting to enlarge the market for electronic information services by encouraging health professionals to search these databases directly. An end user is defined as the person with the information need. Thus, end-user searching is database searching performed by the person who actually needs the information, rather than by a librarian or other search intermediary.

In response to the trend toward end-user systems, librarians are rethinking and redesigning their roles vis-à-vis online searching. Evidence of this change is found in the professional literature in discussions of the impact of end users on librarians and library services[1-3] and in studies that improve our understanding of the characteristics and experiences of end users.[4-7] Librarians have also used the literature as a medium for reviewing and evaluating end-user systems, demonstrating a new consumer advocacy role for the profession.[8-10] Librarians have been particularly concerned with the development and evaluation of end-user training.[11-18] But, as

This chapter was first published in *Medical Reference Services Quarterly*, Vol. 8(3), Fall 1989.

Julia Sollenberger and Bernie Todd Smith point out, teaching computer searching is both labor-intensive and time-consuming.[19] To ensure the best use of limited staff resources, librarians need to establish the extent to which this training effort is worthwhile. What evidence is there that training is related to the end user's ability to search databases effectively?

END-USER SURVEY

This chapter uses data from a general survey of end users to explore the relationship between training and the implementation of end-user searching. In the study, measurement of implementation level reflected a number of different aspects of the amount and quality of online database use. The initial phase of the research involved a case study of a Canadian Medical Association (CMA) pilot test of physician database use through Telecom Canada's iNet 2000 gateway (n = 24). Data from the case study assisted in the design of the questionnaire that was mailed to 150 early adopters of end-user searching in 1986. The questionnaire used as a basis for the results reported here is available upon request from the author.

Many sources were used to identify health professionals who were doing their own database searches. Participants in the CMA pilot project were included, as well as participants in several other trial projects sponsored by hospitals and medical schools. Members of the Canadian Health Libraries Association (CHLA) provided names of end users in their own institutions, and the Canada Institute for Scientific and Technical Information (CISTI) sent the questionnaire to individual subscribers to the U.S. National Library of Medicine's (NLM) MEDLARS databases in Canada. The response rate for the questionnaire was 83 percent.

TRAINING METHODS

The respondents used a variety of methods to become familiar with online searching as shown in Table 13.1. Three-quarters of the end users consulted printed manuals, although only 58.5 percent

TABLE 13.1. Rating of Training Methods

TRAINING METHOD	Not Useful	Somewhat Useful	Very Useful	Total
Printed Manuals (76%)+	13.8 (13)*	28.7 (27)	58.5 (55)	100.0 (94)
Informal Demonstration (45%)	8.9 (5)	41.0 (23)	50.0 (28)	100.0 (56)
Course or Workshop (40%)	4.0 (2)	34.7 (17)	61.2 (30)	100.0 (49)
Online Instruction or Help (35%)	20.5 (9)	25.0 (11)	54.5 (24)	100.0 (44)

* Numbers of respondents are in parentheses.
+ Percent of respondents who reported using each training method.

(n = 55) rated these training aids as "very useful." Informal demonstrations from colleagues, database vendors, or librarians represented the next most common training method (45 percent, n = 56). The large percentage of respondents who rated this method as only "somewhat useful" (41 percent, n = 23) suggests that there is considerable variability in the quality of these informal sessions. Nevertheless, many end users reported using these demonstrations as a learning method. In the study, 73 percent (n = 91) of the respondents reported that they knew at least one other health professional who was doing his or her own database searching. This finding indicates the important part played by an individual's social network of colleagues in the adoption and implementation of new technologies.

Forty percent (n = 49) of the end users reported having taken a course or workshop. This training method received the fewest "not useful" ratings (4 percent, n = 2), in contrast to online instruction and system help which was rated as "not useful" by 20.5 percent (n = 9) of its users. Although the relatively low use of online assistance (35 percent, n = 44) is not surprising to those familiar with the habits of end users, it is still a matter of concern. The considerable resources put into the development of online help systems are wasted if the help is not used. Furthermore, the online environment appears to be the logical place to provide current information on constantly changing databases and search software. Clearly, more exploration is required into the factors related to the usage of online instruction and help, and into methods of making these aids more useful.

Since end users are paying for online connect time, the use of help systems may present a particular problem in this environment. The time-saving nature of online information retrieval is frequently stated in vendor advertising. Not surprisingly, therefore, end users in this study viewed one of the purposes of online searching as saving time. Many users expressed surprise and discouragement at the time it took to become familiar with the online search process. When they accessed an online system, health professionals wanted to use their time and money to produce results (i.e., to find the information they needed) rather than to learn how to use the system. If this situation is typical among end users, then there will be a continuing need for printed manuals and courses. New database storage mediums such as CD-ROM may prove to be more acceptable to users as combined learning and searching tools since there are no online connect charges involved.

MEASURING IMPLEMENTATION

One of the challenges facing researchers in end-user searching is to find an adequate measure of the implementation of end-user searching. Once such a measure is established, the researcher can examine the relationship between the level of implementation and a variety of characteristics of the users and their environments. Researchers studying the diffusion of innovations frequently use the decision to adopt an innovation as the outcome of interest. In the case of online database searching, the adoption-decision point can be defined as the act of signing up for an online system or performing an end-user search for the first time.

A problem with end-user searching, as well as some other so-called intellectual technologies, is that initial interest and use does not guarantee continuing use. End-user searching is an optional activity for most health professionals and the novelty can wear off. In the Canadian Medical Association pilot project that preceded this study, online connect time dipped substantially after the first three months.[20] The previously cited studies of Poisson,[21] and Starr and Renford[22] also show that even health professionals who are committed enough to take an end-user searching course do not necessarily sign up for an online system or become frequent searchers.

In this study, 13 different questions related to the implementation of end-user searching were asked, and a score was calculated for each health professional. High-level implementers of end-user searching were expected to score higher than low-level implementers on the following measures: number of databases searched; number of locations where online databases could be accessed (e.g., office and home); number of others shown how to search; ownership of hardware; frequency of searching; time and money spent on searching; personal payment for searches; willingness to recommend searching to colleagues; complexity of search topics; number of connect hours; and length of searching experience.

Although none of the 13 items is, in itself, a full measure of implementation, the composite provides a reasonable basis for assessment. A reliability analysis of the items showed that the implementation items could be added up to form a single measure (Cronbach's alpha = .72).[23] The respondents showed substantial differences in implementation levels as measured by this scale. The scores ranged from 17 to 36 with a mean of 27 (S.D. 4.59). The minimum possible score was 13 and the maximum possible was 39. These results show that there are considerable differences among end users in searching ability and experience which librarians should keep in mind.

TRAINING AND IMPLEMENTATION

For librarians and others involved in the provision of end-user training, the obvious question is whether training is related to higher implementation levels. In this study, there was a positive association between the total number of training events reported

and the level of implementation (r = .32, p 0.01). The various types
of training reported are shown in Table 13.1. Several types of training, both formal and informal, were related to implementation behavior.

The relationship between taking an end-user training course and
implementation level was not so straightforward. This cross-sec-
tional study included a number of long-time end users who had
begun searching before end-user training courses were available.
These end users were among the highest-level implementers. One of
the perceptual variables measured in the study was called accessibility and control. This variable measured the extent to which respondents valued the extra accessibility to online systems and the personal
control over the search process offered by end-user searching. The
earliest end users, those who had not taken courses, had significantly
higher personal accessibility and control scores (t = 2.89, p < 0.01).
This result suggests that the earliest adopters were more likely to be
independent learners and innovators who were sufficiently motivated
to use online systems despite a lack of formal training opportunities.

Online training courses have been offered on a periodic basis in
major centers for many years. Training on the National Library of
Medicine's MEDLARS system in Canada was initially offered as a
three-day training program by the Canada Institute for Scientific
and Technical Information (CISTI). These courses were originally
intended for search intermediaries. Apparently, the time commitment, as well as the detailed content, discouraged the earliest adopters of end-user searching from attending courses. Recently, training
programs specifically geared to the needs of end users have begun
to emerge. But since it is the more recent adopters of end-user
searching who are taking these courses, the implementation means
of this group are actually lower than those of the earlier adopters
who did not take courses (t = 2.94, p < 0.01).

MEDICAL SUBJECT HEADINGS (MeSH) USE

The use of MeSH, the list of subject terms developed and maintained by the National Library of Medicine, is considered essential
for achieving optimal search results on MEDLINE. Eighty percent

(n = 99) of the end users in this study were searching MEDLINE. The Boolean combination of MeSH terms, with attached subheadings where appropriate, usually produces search results with the highest recall and precision. Large sections of the hierarchical *Tree Structures* of MeSH terms can also be included in a search through the use of explosions. There are times when it is important to search using Text Words, or words that appear in the title or abstract of an article. For instance, this approach is necessary when a topic is too new to have become an official MeSH term.

There is concern among librarians that end users may rely too heavily on the Text Word search capability even when appropriate MeSH terminology is available. End users may not know how to use MeSH or may not recognize the added value of using MeSH terms. In their advertising, database vendors frequently stress the ease of online searching which usually means taking a Text Word approach. Since it is difficult to include all of the potentially relevant synonyms or related concepts in a Text Word search, the results may well be incomplete. The interpretation of the results can also be problematic if the user believes that all of the relevant articles in the database were retrieved using Text Words. Given the concerns of search intermediaries, one purpose of this study was to explore the use of MeSH by health professionals.

If the concerns of librarians and search intermediaries are warranted, the researcher would expect to find some evidence that MeSH use was related to the level of implementation achieved by end users. In the study, 79 percent (n = 98) of the respondents were aware that MeSH existed, although only 53 percent said they use it "very often" or "somewhat often." The remaining 47 percent were apparently continuing to search and retrieve citations from MEDLINE in a reasonably satisfactory way without the sophisticated searching capabilities provided by MeSH use. How did almost half of these end users get along without using MeSH? Possibly, infrequent MeSH users were satisfied with very basic searches and were not able or willing to exert the additional effort required to use the vocabulary terms. Another possibility is that the end users were searching in a limited subject area in which they were already familiar with the MeSH terminology and could therefore use it without consulting the thesaurus. Techniques such as "citation pearl-growing,'' or building a search strategy on the basis of MeSH terms found in the first few relevant records from an initial Text Word search, may have been employed by end users. In any case, there appears to be a substantial number of end users who get along well enough without using MeSH.

Even though MeSH users and nonusers were satisfied enough with their results to continue searching, the actual search results obtained by the two groups may still have been qualitatively different. Continuing to use an innovation such as online searching may not be the same as achieving optimal results. The relationship between MeSH use and a group of variables measuring the respondents' perceptions of end-user searching sheds additional light on this possibility. A comparison of MeSH users and nonusers showed that users generally perceived end-user searching in more positive terms ($t = 2.78$, $p < 0.01$). In particular, MeSH users reported less difficulty in meeting their patient care information needs through online searching than did nonusers ($t = 2.74$, $p < 0.01$).

When frequency of MeSH use was employed as a continuous variable in the analysis, there was a positive relationship between frequency of MeSH use and the following:

1. overall positive perceptions of end-user searching ($r = .26$, $p < 0.01$);
2. perceived relative advantage of end-user searching over previous ways of searching for information ($r = .31$, $p < 0.01$);
3. perceived ability of end-user searching to meet professional information needs ($r = .36$, $p < 0.01$); and
4. perceived usefulness of end-user searching as an innovation ($r = .33$, $p < 0.01$).

Although these correlations should not be interpreted in a causal manner, they do provide some evidence that frequency of MeSH use is associated with more positive perceptions of end-user searching. Further analysis of the study data revealed that end users' perceptions of online searching explained or predicted up to 46 percent of their implementation levels. Thus, a link was made between MeSH use and end users' perceptions of online searching which, in turn, predicted implementation levels.

CONCLUSION

The results of this study provide some preliminary empirical evidence that training does make a difference to the implementation of end-user searching. The total number of training events reported, including training opportunities of both a formal and informal nature, was positively correlated with implementation level. Furthermore, MeSH users were found to have more positive perceptions of end-user searching than nonusers. More positive perceptions of end-user searching were, in turn, predictive of higher implementation levels.

There are several implications of these findings for future end-user training efforts. First, because end users were found to vary in their implementation levels, librarians should remain attuned to the differences among end users and resist the temptation to think of end users as a single homogeneous group. Training that takes into account different professional backgrounds, subject interests, and varying levels of expertise in online searching will be required in the future.

Since the total number of training events–not simply having taken a formal end-user course–was correlated with implementation, librarians would be wise to take a broad view of what constitutes end-user training. Informal demonstrations and discussions with end users are often the best "teachable moments." Librarians have instinctively done this kind of informal teaching for a long time without any special recognition; however, this study gives support to its importance as a component of the total training effort. Since a lot of informal teaching goes on among end users themselves, the impact of the single librarian/end user interaction is multiplied. The results also indicate that there are end users who can get along quite well without formal training opportunities. There may be imaginative ways that librarians can take advantage of the end-user social network to enlarge teaching and support capabilities within an institution or local area.

Finally, these results confirm the importance of continuing to teach the use of MeSH. The data show clearly that the use of MeSH is related to the value placed on online searching by health professionals accessing MEDLINE and the other MEDLARS databases which use the MeSH vocabulary. Librarians have recognized the value of MeSH for many years and have included it in training programs. Fortunately, MeSH use is now becoming easier for end users with front-end programs such as Grateful MED and some of the CD-ROM products that provide access to MeSH vocabulary.

For health sciences librarians and information specialists who are in close touch with end users, some of the results reported here may not be news. Several of the hypotheses were designed to test conventional wisdom that has existed in the field for some years. Nevertheless, the profession needs to gather and present observable evidence to confirm or disconfirm commonly accepted beliefs and individual experience. Exploring issues such as the relationship between training and the implementation of end-user searching also reveals the complexity of some of the research questions in the field. There is a need for further development of models and measurement instruments that can assist librarians to explore these questions in greater depth.

REFERENCES

1. Ojala, Marydee. "End User Searching and Its Implications for Librarians." *Special Libraries* 76 (Spring 1985):93-99.

2. Olmsted, Marcia. "The End User and the Librarian: Perspectives from a DIALOG Trainer." *Canadian Library Journal* 43 (February 1986):49-53.

3. Shedlock, James. "Planning for End User Services in the Health Sciences Library." *Medical Reference Services Quarterly* 6 (Winter 1987):1-13.

4. Marshall, Joanne Gard. "Characteristics of Early Adopters of End-User Online Searching in the Health Professions." *Bulletin of the Medical Library Association* 77 (January 1989):48-55.

5. Roberts, Justine, and Jensen, Lydia. "Self-Service at the Information Supermarket: Report on an End User's Online ShoppingTrip." *Reference Librarian* 16 (Winter 1986):153-175.

6. St. Jacques, Suzanne. "End-User Searching for a Large Student Clientele at the University of Ottawa: Where We've Been, Where We Are, Where We're Going." *Canadian Journal of Information Science* 11(3/4, 1986):122-130.

7. Sewell, Winifred, and Teitlebaum, Sandra. "Observations of End-User Online Searching Behavior Over Eleven Years." *Journal of the American Society for Information Science* 37 (July 1986):234-245.

8. Bonham, Miriam D., and Nelson, Laurie L. "An Evaluation of Four End-User Systems for Searching MEDLINE." *Bulletin of the Medical Library Association* 76 (January 1988):22-31.

9. Homan, J. Michael. "End-User Information Utilities in the Health Sciences." *Bulletin of the Medical Library Association* 74 (January 1986):31-35.

10. Marshall, Joanne Gard. "How to Choose the Online Medical Database That's Right for You." *Canadian Medical Association Journal* 134 (March 15, 1986):634-640.

11. Cheney, Paul H., and Nelson, R. Ryan. "A Tool for Measuring and Analysing End User Computing Abilities." *Information Processing and Management* 24 (1988):199-203.

12. Ginn, David S.; Pinkowski, Patricia E.; and Tylman, Wieslawa T. "Evolution of an End-User Training Program." *Bulletin of the Medical Library Association* 75 (April 1987):117-121.

13. Haines, Judith S. "Experiences in Training End-User Searchers." *Online* 6 (November 1982):14-23.

14. Penhale, Sara J., and Taylor, Nancy. "Integrating End-User Searching into a Bibliographic Instruction Program." *RQ* 27 (Winter 1986):212-220.

15. Poisson, Ellen H. "End-User Searching in Medicine." *Bulletin of the Medical Library Association* 74 (October 1986):293-299.

16. Snow, Bonnie. "Making the Rough Places Plain: Designing MEDLINE End User Training." *Medical Reference Services Quarterly* 3 (Winter 1984):1-11.

17. Starr, Susan S., and Renford, Beverly L. "Evaluation of a Program to Teach Health Professionals to Search MEDLINE." *Bulletin of the Medical Library Association* 75 (July 1987):193-201.

18. Welborn, Victoria, and Kuehn, Jennifer J. "End-User Programs in Medical School Libraries: A Survey." *Bulletin of the Medical Library Association* 76 (January 1988):137-140.

19. Sollenberger, Julia, and Smith, Bernie Todd. "Teaching Computer Searching to Health Care Professionals: Why Does It Take So Long?" *Medical Reference Services Quarterly* 6 (Winter 1987):45-51.

20. Marshall, Joanne Gard; Banner, Sandra; and Chouinard, Joseph L. *Physicians Online: Final Report of the CMA iNet Trial.* Ottawa: Canadian Medical Association, 1986.

21. Poisson, p. 296.

22. Starr and Renford, p. 193.

23. Babbie, Earl. *The Practice of Social Research.* 4th ed. Belmont: Wadsworth, 1986, 526-527.

Chapter 14

End-User Searching
and New Roles for Librarians

Barbara Lowther Shipman
Diane G. Schwartz
Sandra C. Dow

INTRODUCTION

Since 1988, the rapid proliferation of databases available to end
users at the University of Michigan (UM) has impacted the role of
librarians dramatically. While librarians at the Taubman Medical
Library (TML) had seen a gradual change in role throughout the
1980s, the last several years launched them into the future.

Michigan has provided access to a number of CD-ROM databases for quite some time. In 1988, the NOTIS-based online catalog, known as MIRLYN, came up. This was the first database
widely available to end users. In early 1989, free unlimited searching of PaperChase (known locally as UM-MEDLINE) was made
available to students, faculty, and staff of the University. Michigan
was one of the first institutions to purchase NOTIS' Multiple Database Access System (MDAS), and, later in 1989, six Wilson indexes and PsycINFO were brought up. Three additional databases
are currently available through MIRLYN.

The introduction of UM-MEDLINE is the best example of how
the roles of librarians have been changing due to the introduction of
electronic information resources. It has had an impact on the impor-

---

This chapter was first published in *Medical Reference Services Quarterly*, Vol.
11(3), Fall 1992.

tance and level of mediated searching, the type of reference questions received, the instructional programs offered, and the role and responsibilities of the database services coordinator. This chapter will describe the changes in role resulting from a massive end-user searching program and the ways in which one library has prepared its staff to deal with them.

START-UP ACTIVITIES

The contract with PaperChase was signed in October 1988, with a target start-up date of January 1989. With a relatively short lead time there was a great deal of preparation to be done. In addition to traditional activities such as developing training programs and handouts and training library staff to search a new system, there were other less traditional things to be done. These included modifying generic screen displays for UM users and learning the PaperChase management functions which allow local management of the system. While PaperChase staff created the online journal holdings list, it was first necessary to match UM's holdings against the list of journal titles indexed for MEDLINE. This was originally thought to be a project that could be handled by student employees. However, due to the number of titles received, the complexity of the serials records, and the nature of the list provided by PaperChase, the project required the skill of a librarian and was the most time-consuming of the start-up activities.

GENERAL IMPACTS

The use of UM-MEDLINE has been phenomenal. Figure 14.1 illustrates the growth in its use since it became available in mid-January 1989. It was used almost 102,000 times in 1989; use increased by 37 percent in 1990, to around 140,000 uses. In 1989, 5,968 people became registered users of UM-MEDLINE, with an additional 3,387 registering in 1990. UM users have logged over 60,500 connect hours online. Although librarians at Taubman had felt some effects of end-user searching for a number of years, no one had anticipated the total impact of this level of use.

The impact of UM-MEDLINE availability on the library was felt immediately, and affected both staff and services. The greatest effect was on the information services staff, who were expected to answer a variety of questions that had previously been handled by one or two staff members. These questions related to computer hardware and software, and required much more specific knowledge than most staff members possessed. In addition, while end users had been provided with information on how to search, this was usually done in relation to systems on which librarians had a great deal of searching experience. With PaperChase, staff had about a month in which to become experts before the questions began. It is very important to anticipate the implications of remote access and end-user searching for public services staff before implementing new systems or planning for staff development.

The second major impact was on the mediated search service. Although searching had been declining since 1986 due to a moderate level of end-user searching of BRS Colleague and Compact

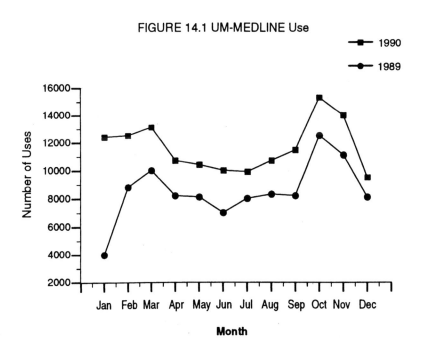

FIGURE 14.1 UM-MEDLINE Use

Cambridge MEDLINE, librarians had sustained a reasonable level of searching. With the availability of UM-MEDLINE, there was an immediate and sharp decrease in mediated searching (see Figure 14.2). This decrease continued for 14 months, then leveled off. The current searchload is only 28 percent of what it was before UM-MEDLINE became available (see Figure 14.3). This decrease in mediated searching has several implications. First, librarians may VVnot be doing enough searching to maintain their search skills. Second, there are not enough incoming searches to allow new searchers to be trained in the same way that they have been in the past. This is a real problem due to ongoing training needs for people in the two-year Research Library Residency and University Library Associates programs. Third, one would expect that librarians would now have available the time that was once spent on searching. This has not proven to be the case. Although librarians are doing fewer searches than in the past, they are spending an average of 10 percent longer per search than they were before PaperChase came up (see Table 14.1). Some of this increase may be because search skills are not as sharp as they once were. The fact that interview times have decreased, while formulation and online times, which are more likely to be affected by skill level, have increased, to some extent confirms this (see Table 14.1). Individual searchers are now doing fewer than half as many searches per year as they were before UM-MEDLINE came up (see Table 14.2). The rise in search time may also be due in part to the growing complexity of searches, which is reflected in the increase in formulation time (see Table 14.1). Although there are some "regular" clients who have never done their own searching, it appears that other clients are bringing librarians those searches which are too complicated to be run in PaperChase. In addition, searchers are now serving as consultants to end users, advising them on search strategy as well as software setup. As users become more experienced online searchers, they begin to ask for more computer support.

IMPACT ON REFERENCE DESK SERVICES

The use of a number of different computer systems by users with greatly varying levels of computer skills has impacted all informa-

FIGURE 14.2. Mediated Online Searches

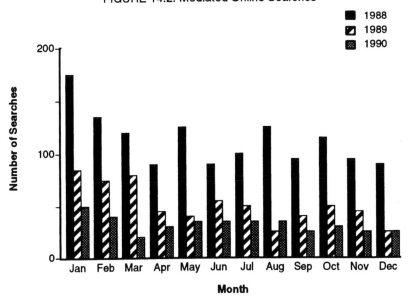

FIGURE 14.3. Decline in Mediated Searching

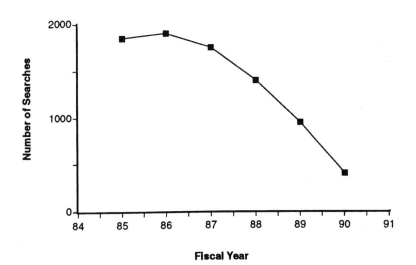

TABLE 14.1. Mediated Searches

	1987	1988	% change	1989	% change	1990	% change
Interview time	6.4	5.8	−9.4	5.7	−1.7	5.5	−3.5
Formulation time	7.8	7.8	0	8.2	+5.1	9.6	+17.1
Online time	21.2	23.0	+8.5	24.3	+5.7	25.2	+3.7
Total time	35.4	36.6	+3.4	38.2	+4.4	40.3	+5.6
Average searches per searcher	203	139	−31.5	67	−51.8	61	−9.0

Note: Time is in minutes.

TABLE 14.2. Average Number of Searches Per Searcher

	Total number of searches	Number of searchers	Average number per searcher
1987	1,624	8	203.0
1988	1,255	9	139.4
1989	601	9	66.8
1990	394	6	60.7

tion services staff. New user demands have caused increased demands on staff. Where in the past it was adequate to concentrate computer and instructional expertise in a few staff members, everyone now needs to be prepared to provide formal and informal instruction on subjects ranging from use of the OPAC to database management software, as well as information on computer hardware and software.

UM-MEDLINE has had a significant impact on activity at the library's reference desk in the past two years. In 1989, the first year of operation, extended reference questions (those requiring more than five minutes to answer) rose by 24 percent when compared to the previous year, while in the second full year of operation, 1990, extended reference questions increased by 40 percent (see Table 14.3). When total reference activity in 1988 is compared to total activity in 1990, there is an 18 percent increase; extended reference activity showed a 73 percent increase for the same time period. Overall there was an increase in total reference activity of 11 percent between 1988 and 1989, while between 1989 and 1990 there was an increase of 7 percent. When total reference activity in 1988 is compared to total reference activity in 1990, an 18 percent increase is noted.

The significant increase in extended reference questions answered reflects the complex issues with which users were confronted when setting up access to UM-MEDLINE. Since UM-MEDLINE is available to users wherever they can connect to the state's MichNet network, its implementation set in motion a complex set of issues that users had to resolve. From its inception, the staff of the Taubman Medical Library had total local responsibility for operating UM-MEDLINE, and users were encouraged to call the library for assistance.

While the Information Services Department has long sought to cover the desk in the afternoons with two staff members, it was not always possible in 1989/90 because of staff reductions. Troubleshooting printer problems, instructing users, and answering traditional reference questions, whether received by telephone or in person, has frequently been the purview of one staff member at a time. To verify the impact being made by the variety of electronic information sources available for public use in the reference area, a new category of question, "electronic," was added to the reference desk statistics form. To ensure consistency in recording activity in this new area, it was defined as "the answer given to any question that dealt with searching UM-MEDLINE, the OPAC, either of the two CD-ROM databases available, or any other computer-related question." Both on-site and telephone queries were recorded. Between April 1990 and December 1991, 18 percent of all reference questions answered fell into this category (see Figure 14.4).

In 1989, the first full year of UM-MEDLINE operation, there was

TABLE 14.3. Reference Questions

Type Of Question	1987	1988	% change	1989	% change	1990	% change
Quick	18,664	20,350	+9.0	21,989	+8.1	22,049	+0.3
Extended	3,634	3,632	−0.1	4,499	+23.9	6,297	+40.0
Telephone	5,694	6,114	+7.3	6,667	+9.0	7,448	+11.7

a 9 percent increase in the number of telephone reference questions answered as compared to the previous year (see Figure 14.5). Many of these calls concerned UM-MEDLINE. Because the new systems have made it possible for users to access the library from their own computers for the first time, it is not unreasonable to assume that increases in telephone queries are related to the availability of remote access to the library. This may, in fact, explain the 24 percent increase in the number of extended reference questions handled in 1989 when compared to the previous year (see Table 14.3).

While many of the changes in activities that have taken place at the reference desk are quantifiable, others are not. For example, in the past during quiet times, staff members would search the OPAC or RLIN in support of their book selection responsibilities. Some staff would catch up on professional reading. Since the advent of UM-MEDLINE, staff have little time for these activities. Staff consistently report, "there is no flexible time at the reference desk these days . . . [and] with all the information [sources] available to library users . . . [via the OPAC, UM-MEDLINE, etc.] the questions they bring to us are more complex."

UM librarians' experience with UM-MEDLINE offers valuable insight that can be useful to others interested in providing access to MEDLINE to a wide audience. First, librarians should plan for an adequate number of workstations close to the reference desk. Although UM-MEDLINE is available for users to search from homes, offices, or laboratories, a significant number of users need the crutch of searching in the library where assistance is available. Second, as many workstations as possible should be installed. TML's initial installation of two dedicated workstations was inadequate and re-

FIGURE 14.4. Average Number of Searches Per Searcher

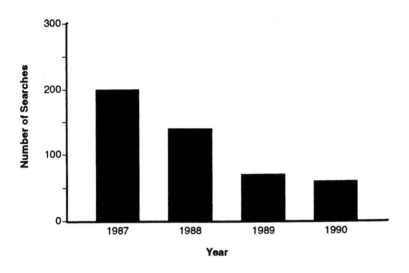

FIGURE 14.5. Reference Questions

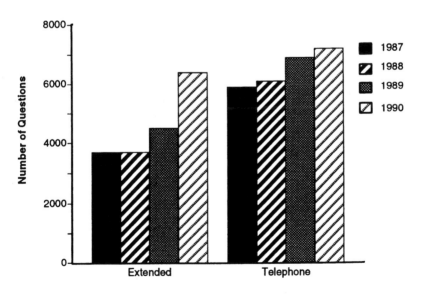

sulted in waiting lines and unhappy users. Even today, with three workstations dedicated to searching UM-MEDLINE, waiting lines are not uncommon. Third, in order to handle increased reference activity, librarians should double staff the reference desk if possible. In September 1990, four new staff members joined the Information Services Division, making it possible to double staff the reference desk on a routine basis. Now that "Electronic" questions have been recorded for over a year, it is interesting to note that a regular increase in the number of questions handled has occurred. As expected, the percent increase was greater during Fall term with the onset of the academic year than in Spring/Summer when activity in the library is usually a bit slower. TML librarians plan to continue to monitor the demand for service in this area and to use that information to determine how best to staff the reference/information desk to provide users with quality service when they need it.

IMPACT ON INSTRUCTIONAL SERVICES

In the first two years that UM-MEDLINE was available, Taubman librarians taught 242 classes to almost 3,000 users, of which 84 percent were hands-on sessions (see Figure 14.6). The total number of classes represents a 40 percent increase in the number of classes taught prior to the introduction of UM-MEDLINE and a 31 percent increase in hands-on sessions. Close to 20 percent of the almost 11,000 registered users at the University have been reached with one of the instructional sessions given by the Medical Library alone (see Figure 14.7). This does not take into account either the numbers taught at the Dentistry, Public Health, or other libraries on campus or people taught one-on-one at the reference desk. In 1989, 28 percent more people were taught than in the previous year, but this increase was not sustained in 1990. Although 40 percent more classes are being taught than in the past, only 20 percent more users are being reached. The demand for more classes is coming from a select group of sophisticated users for highly specialized sessions.

A new instructional problem was staff training. Reference staff were now required to teach users the basics of searching Paper-Chase, and they also had to develop expertise in the area of technical support. Taubman staff were required to become familiar with a

FIGURE 14.6. Classes Taught

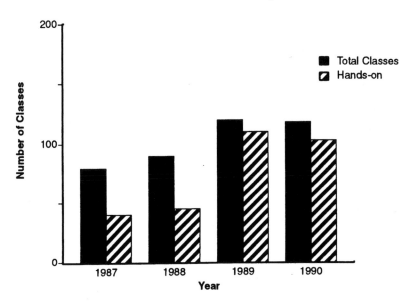

FIGURE 14.7. Number of People Taught in Formal Classes

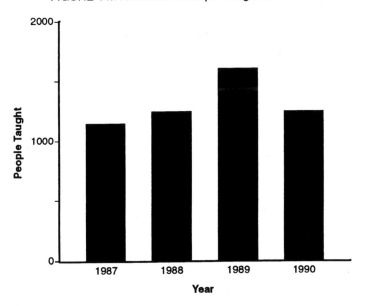

number of different telecommunications software packages in order to help users configure their software properly and tell them how to activate their printers as well as the disk drive for downloading. A software problem-solving handout was developed which could be used for answering these questions and for distribution to users.

After a year of unlimited access to UM-MEDLINE, librarians noticed an increase in the number of questions relating to database management software. Librarians had offered hands-on instructional sessions on Pro-Cite for three years, but users began asking for information about other database management software. Because librarians did not want to promote one package over others, a new instructional session was developed to demonstrate a variety of database management packages. The purpose of the session was to allow users to see the programs in action. Several handouts were also developed which outlined advantages and disadvantages of the programs as well as system requirements. As a result of the preparation required for this session, Taubman now has staff experts who can answer users' questions about a number of programs. An immediate result of this session has been a demand for instructional sessions on most of the packages demonstrated.

Implementing UM-MEDLINE has necessitated the development of instructional skills for all information services librarians. At the same time, librarians had to develop a broader understanding of users' needs, including how to identify and fulfill them. The development of increasing expectations and sophistication of database end users has required librarians to scramble in an effort to stay on top of this rapidly developing technology in order to retain their leadership role. Simultaneously librarians must respond quickly to users' perceived needs; if not, users will seek assistance elsewhere.

MANAGEMENT OF DATABASE SEARCH SERVICES

The advent of a major end-user search program and all the attendant administrative responsibilities, along with the decline in mediated searching, have resulted in a major change in role for the database services coordinator. The traditional job responsibilities for this position included monitoring the quality of searching, which was a time-consuming process; training new searchers for mediated searching, which could take from three to 12 months; overseeing staff equipment and troubleshooting problems; recommending new vendors and databases for access; and staying abreast of developments in the field of online searching. These traditional responsibilities have all changed to some extent. Monitoring the quality of searching is no longer very time-consuming, due to the decreased number of searches being done (see Figure 14.2). Conversely, training new searchers has become quite a lengthy process due to the lack of new searches to work on. Working on actual current searches has been supplanted by reworking old searches on paper, which does not develop interviewing skills (although trainees may now have more opportunity to develop these skills at the reference desk). In addition to the six staff microcomputers in information services, there are now eight public access computers that require regular troubleshooting. And while staying abreast of new developments in the field was once confined to online searching, it has now been expanded to include computer hardware, software, and networking.

As end users master UM-MEDLINE, demand for additional database services increases. New responsibilities for the database services coordinator include evaluating and recommending new products and services, such as CD-ROMs, and diskette-based and networked products, as well as determining ways of adapting existing products to the local environment. This can require working closely with systems people, which necessitates more knowledge of the mainframe and client-server environments than was needed in the past. The coordinator's knowledge of databases and search systems has been put to use in an increasing involvement in writing specifications for new systems and services, and negotiating with vendors to design and implement systems that meet unique local needs.

It is no longer adequate that information services staff be trained online searchers. In order to serve as credible consultants to end-user searchers, librarians must be able to deal with a wide variety of computer-related questions, many of which are asked by people with little or no knowledge of computers. It is the responsibility of the database services coordinator to ensure that staff can serve in this new role as consultant to both novice and expert computer users by providing computer literacy training, as well as traditional training in online searching. The traditional training in searching remains important: it is difficult for someone who is not an expert searcher to advise a user on how to formulate a search. An additional problem to be dealt with is how to maintain search skills when there are few searches to work on. However, for consulting, knowledge of the MEDLINE database is proving more important than use of any one command language to search it.

The daily local management of PaperChase has resulted in additional responsibilities that further changed the role of the database services coordinator. Although this position has always served as the vendor liaison, this role becomes much more important when it affects the whole University community, rather than one department. It has been very important to build and maintain a close working relationship with PaperChase staff. The identification of system and network problems also becomes more critical when problems affect so many local users. The coordinator has worked closely with the vendor to customize screen displays and options for local use. A major new responsibility relates to PaperChase's online comment capability, which lets users leave comments and questions. In order to encourage users to identify PaperChase access with the library, librarians respond to these comments and questions. Users do in fact identify PaperChase access with the library, and library staff, especially those providing responses, are widely recognized as the experts. The database services coordinator also oversees the validation and entry of new users who are not yet in the database of PaperChase users. This further reinforces the role of the library as central to the functioning of PaperChase.

In sum, the database services coordinator now manages a search service with thousands of searchers, rather than only eight. Some of the job responsibilities that once related to mediated searching must in the future be applied to end-user searching, in particular evaluating the service and the quality of the work being done.

CONCLUSION

The availability of unlimited free access to the MEDLINE database at the University of Michigan has done more to enhance the role of the medical librarian than has anything else since online searching first became available here in the early 1970s. The role that the library has taken in the management of UM-MEDLINE, and the decisions that were made to handle locally all problems and questions associated with it, have served to identify library staff as experts to all who use the database. Due to the widespread use of UM-MEDLINE and other locally available databases, reference librarians are now teaching people how to search as often as they are finding answers to questions. Where it was once enough to have one or two staff members capable of responding to technical questions relating to hardware and software, it is now necessary for all information services staff to be able to respond to these questions if users are to be provided with adequate service. Where searchers once used their knowledge of online searching to provide clients with searches, they are now using this knowledge to advise users on how to do their own searches. Where the database services coordinator once administered a service providing searches to around 2,000 people a year, she now administers a service used by 2,000 to 3,000 people a month. The knowledge of online searching acquired over a number of years is being applied as a knowledge of online retrieval systems and database structure. This type of knowledge is applicable in any number of areas in the current environment, and complements the knowledge of systems staff and programmers, with whom librarians will more and more often find themselves working closely. The possibilities seem endless.

As librarians develop new skills and a broader understanding of users' needs, it becomes increasingly important to stay one step ahead of users in order to respond quickly to their perceived needs. If librarians fail to take on the challenge, users may go elsewhere for their information management needs. If librarians are successful, the enhanced skill and expertise acquired will be met with greater user recognition and appreciation of the role of medical librarians.

PART III
RESEARCH IN USER EDUCATION

Chapter 15

Reflections on Educational Research Needed in Special Libraries

Martha Jane K. Zachert

INTRODUCTION

The literature of occupational groups which call themselves professionals typically progresses from descriptions of personal or institutional experience to empirical research to theoretical formulations. The general literature produced by health sciences and other special librarians follows this pattern. Descriptions and tips to improve performance come first. Then experience is converted to hypotheses which are tested and from which conclusions are drawn. After rival hypotheses have been tested, replicated, and enhanced, theories are formulated. Such studied principles provide the foundation for long periods of practice.

Most of the literature about group instruction in special libraries is in the first stage of this progression. A recent study of articles published over a 15-year period showed that 70 percent of these articles are descriptions of experience in a single library.[1] Another 10.5 percent are reviews of literature or descriptions of multilibrary experiences. The latter are usually the result of introductory surveys. Reports of empirical or theoretical research are noticeably lacking.

The initial study of health sciences library literature, described above, was extended to include published reports from other special

This chapter was first published in *Medical Reference Services Quarterly*, Vol. 10(1), Spring 1991.

libraries, especially legal, corporate, and government libraries.[2] As expected, the same paucity of research and emphasis on description was evident. More important, both studies led to two significant observations:

1. There are four target audiences for educational services in libraries. In numbers of learners, library users are the largest group. However, library staff, library school students, and professional peers also constitute significant audiences for library-sponsored instruction.[3]
2. Educational services in special libraries are an expanding trend, vigorous, innovative, and ready for research.

This chapter will suggest questions for empirical study in four areas: (1) the assumptions underlying educational services; (2) aspects of management of this type of work; (3) pedagogical considerations to achieve the best possible cost-benefit ratio; and (4) new modes of evaluation to elicit information that will benefit management of group teaching and improve educational effectiveness.

ASSUMPTIONS UNDERLYING INSTRUCTION

Several assumptions have been stated in the literature of library instruction, and operational decisions are based on them. In spite of the 15 or more years during which instructional services have been growing in special libraries, these assumptions are still untested. Instructional programs require the expenditure of so many resources that every assumption needs to be examined carefully and, if at all possible, tested empirically. The research questions are: Are these assumptions valid? Do the variations known to exist in different special library environments affect this validity? If so, how?

The following are especially significant assumptions being used in decision making about library instruction:

1. Ultimate costs of total library service are lowered by some degree of user self-sufficiency.
2. Ultimate costs of total library service are lowered and high

quality is maintained by staff instruction, both initial job training and continuing education.
3. Participation in the educational programs of professional
associations is mutually beneficial when a library permits its
staff to serve as teachers in those programs.
4. After library instruction, student users of academic special
libraries learn more effectively in all of their course work.
5. After library instruction, the professionals who are the special
library's users perform their work more effectively.

Considerable attention is being focused on how to present
instruction. It is important not to forget, while concentrating on the
logistics of educational activities, that a solid foundation of research
is significant for decision making. Knowledge about the validity of
these and other assumptions would provide a surer footing than is
presently available.

MANAGEMENT OF EDUCATIONAL SERVICES

Those special libraries which are committed to educational services have found different ways to organize their staffs for service.
The patterns most frequently found in the author's analysis are the
following:

1. One member of a department (usually reference or information service) is assigned to be "education librarian" and carries out all aspects of the service.
2. An "education coordinator" is appointed to direct the service
by delegating various related tasks to qualified staff from
throughout the library organization.
3. A separate education department is established, with its own
director and, sometimes, additional teaching librarians and
support staff. This department may use staff from throughout
the library for specialized purposes.[4]

Whichever pattern is chosen, the relationships between organizational pattern, program acceptance, and cost-benefit need to be studied. Is one organizational pattern superior in some aspect? Is any

given pattern preferable in a given library environment? What are the advantages or disadvantages of each organizational arrangement? Comparative cost studies of these and other possible patterns are also needed.

All aspects of financing educational services need study; the variations are too numerous to state here. Of special concern should be the application to educational services of overhead formulas devised for use in relation to other library services.[5] Are such formulas valid for educational services budgets?

Personnel costs typically represent the major investment in a library's educational services program, and the relationship between personnel effectiveness and program success is obvious. All aspects of personnel management each with its own questions should, therefore, be the subject of research. Since this area is less well represented in the descriptive literature than others, factual studies from different library environments are needed to precede comparative studies.[6]

The success or failure and the cost-benefit ratio of library educational services may well depend on the ways in which they are marketed.[7] It is critical to ask: Which marketing schemes are most persuasive? Is success dependent on library environment or target audience? Are formal marketing procedures worth their cost?

PEDAGOGICAL CONSIDERATIONS

What motivates adult learners in audiences targeted by libraries? Which learning styles do these learners prefer? Which teaching styles are most productive for them? Can preferred learning styles be accommodated in typical library instructional designs? Can library teachers adapt to learners' preferred styles without adding unduly to the cost of instruction? The cost/benefit implication of answers to these questions is apparent.[8] Here the literature of general adult education, if used with caution, can help to formulate hypotheses.[9] Having discovered what one can about applicable motivational methods and learning-teaching styles, research could proceed to the testing of alternative instructional designs and their comparative costs.[10]

EVALUATION OF EDUCATIONAL PROGRAMS

Evaluation, arguably the most important part of the administration of educational programs, suffers from a lack of focus, rigor, consistency over time, and objectivity. Improved methods could be developed (or borrowed from other disciplines) and tested in the library instructional environment. More general questions should then be addressed. Are services appropriate to objectives? Are selected management techniques effective? What resources are required to obtain various benefits? What, exactly, are the learning and other outcomes of the distinctive educational work done in special libraries?[11]

IS THERE STILL A NEED
FOR DESCRIPTIVE LITERATURE?

Indeed, there is still a need for descriptive literature! Descriptions of educational services in some library environments are especially needed for the preparation of hypotheses for empirical study. For example, the experience of small special libraries and of nonhealth sciences libraries in nonacademic settings is underrepresented in the literature. All kinds of libraries and all kinds of educational services need continuing descriptive reporting to lead to accurate state-of-the-art reviews of practice. The broader the base of such reviews, the more productive the hypotheses developed from them. Marketing, as a newer, less-used adjunct of program management, needs both more descriptive literature *and* empirical research.

What are the long-term outcomes of educational services? This is a different question from that of immediate outcomes of specific events. Its implications for both the costs and the benefits of educational services are extremely significant. To answer this critical question, descriptive literature about long-term outcomes of programs in various types of special libraries is needed first. Then empirical studies can be formulated.

IS THEORETICAL RESEARCH NEEDED?

Of course theoretical research is needed eventually. Library instruction is a recent development in special libraries, with the exception of bibliographic instruction in academic special libraries. Outside the academic world, bibliographic instruction is less often offered; rather, the educational offerings address different needs, usually in very different presentational modes. Academic-style bibliographic instruction has a large literature of its own, including numerous research reports from which a number of theories have been developed. Nonacademic special libraries need to move from description to empirical research to the development of theory. This is the progression now needed for special libraries outside the academic world.

CONCLUSION

One might ask, "Why bother with research if educational services are going well?" Information resulting from research will enable special librarians to make well-informed decisions either to invest their resources in educational services or to use them for other purposes. Justification to management about educational services will carry greater conviction if based on research. In other words, the most important reason for this kind of operational research is to facilitate good management decisions. Other benefits, such as the development of theories, are a bonus.

NOTES

1. Zachert, M.J.K. "Educational Services in Health Sciences Libraries: An Analysis of the Literature, 1975-86." *Bulletin of the Medical Library Association* 75 (July 1987):234-238.

2. Zachert, M.J.K. *Educational Services in Special Libraries: Planning and Administration.* Chicago: Medical Library Association, 1990.

3. *Ibid.*, pp. 3-5.

4. *Ibid.*, pp. 117-121.

5. *Ibid.*, p. 151.

6. *Ibid.*, pp. 21-28.

7. *Ibid.*, pp. 187-189,194-195.

8. *Ibid.*, pp. 19-22.

9. Cross, K.P. *Adults as Learners.* San Francisco: Jossey-Bass Publishers, 1981. See especially Chapters 3-6, pp. 50-151.

10. See examples of classic and innovative instructional methods in Zachert, *Educational Services in Special Libraries,* Chapters 4 and 5 and their accompanying case studies, pp. 57-94.

11. *Ibid.*, pp. 149-169.

Chapter 16

User Education
in Academic Health Sciences Libraries:
Results of a Survey

Phyllis C. Self

It is a curious paradox that instruction in library use, which so
many librarians regard as one of the highest forms of library
service, remains so ill-defined and poorly organized. The
teaching function is claimed to be important in determining
our status, but we appear to take this responsibility lightly or
even to neglect it.[1]

INTRODUCTION

In the early 1930s a questionnaire was sent to 54 medical
schools. Only one of the 47 responding schools reported that library
instruction was given by a librarian and was a required course. In
many other schools, lectures or demonstrations were given by
librarians or professors, but attendance was strictly voluntary.[2]
There was, however, active interest in user education in the U.S. as
well as abroad. Since that time, user education has become a topic
of discussion at national and international conferences and within
the professional literature.

In 1980, the American Library Association adopted "Policy

This chapter was first published in *Medical Reference Services Quarterly*, Vol.
9(4), Winter 1990.

Statement: Instruction in the Use of Libraries." It summarizes the issues and outlines goals for librarians in the 1980s. Its final statement served as a motivating force for this research project.

> It is essential that libraries of all types accept the responsibility of providing people with opportunities to understand the organization of information. The responsibility of educating users in successful information location demands the same administrative, funding, and staffing support as do more traditional library programs.[3]

Managing a large academic health sciences library is difficult. Faced with limited budgets and growing user expectations, even the most resourceful individuals are confronted with demands that cannot be met. Traditionally, every effort has been made to protect library collections. Moving from manual to electronic information systems, today's managers must not only continue to protect collections and automate library operations, but offer a wider range of educational programs than ever before with little to no increase in budgets.

In order to examine the issues of administration, funding, and staffing support of user education programs in academic health sciences libraries, a questionnaire was mailed to academic health sciences library directors. The questionnaire was based on the Association of College and Research Libraries (ACRL) Bibliographic Instruction Task Force's 1977 *Guidelines for Bibliographic Instruction in Academic Libraries*. These *Guidelines* were developed "in order to assist college and university libraries in the planning and evaluation of effective programs to instruct members of the academic community in the identification and use of information resources."[4]

METHOD

In this study, the current status of user education is examined in terms of organizational structures and program offerings. Organizational structures for user education included the following categories:

- separate department
- discrete entity within the reference division
- responsibility of audiovisual experts
- function of subject specialists or bibliographers
- potpourri of talented staff drawn from many areas
- coordinator specially selected to work with all library units
- other categories identified by respondents in the study.

A questionnaire was mailed to all members of the Association of Academic Health Sciences Library Directors (AAHSLD) to obtain data which would be useful to those libraries interested in comparing management characteristics, such as organizational structures and types of program offerings. The categories of user education organization structures were taken from the work of George, Hogan, and Beaubien.[5]

The categories for instructional programs (Grateful MED, enduser searching, etc.) were developed from input from several user education providers. The questionnaire was pretested on three library directors and three user education providers. A revised questionnaire was mailed to each member of AAHSLD (117 questionnaires) in late 1988.

RESULTS

Three of the 117 questionnaires were returned with explanations for nonparticipation; 87 were returned with usable data, for a response rate of 76.3 percent. Most respondents reported that they had no written profile of their community's information needs (78.6 percent) nor a written statement of user educational objectives serving as a guide for all user education programs within their institution (74.4 percent).

Education Objectives

Of the 22 respondents who reported having user education objectives, 68.2 percent reported that the academic community is involved with the formulation of immediate objectives, and 63.6 percent of the respondents involve the academic community in setting long-range objectives. Libraries involve the academic community more frequently in evaluating individual user education programs (84.6 percent) than in evaluating the total education program (34.6 percent). Seventy-two percent of the respondents evaluated the effectiveness of the instructional programs in terms of its written objectives. The method used most frequently to evaluate educational programs against written objectives was participant evaluation forms. Other methods included annual reviews, focus groups, questionnaires prior to each class, retreats, comments from staff and users, and user surveys.

Organizational Structures

A variety of organizational structures exist through which user education programs may be provided. There may be a separate user education department, a part of a larger division, a potpourri of staff from many areas, subject specialists or bibliographers, or a coordinator for user education. The majority of respondents indicated that user education librarians are not clearly identifiable in the organizational chart nor do they hold a status similar to persons responsible for planning, implementing, and evaluating the other major functions of the library, such as the head of reference services. The majority of respondents reported that individuals responsible for user education report to either the head of reference services (31.0 percent) or the library director (31.0 percent); only 17.2 percent report to a coordinator. Almost half of the respondents (47.2 percent) agreed that the organization for user education activities will continue, 28.7 percent were uncertain, and 24.1 percent believed the organization may change in the next five years.

Location

User education takes place primarily in the library (86, or 98.9 percent) followed by an academic faculty member's classroom (57, or 65.5 percent). The least used area for instruction is the hospital. Only 22 (25.3 percent) reported some use of hospital facilities for instruction. A number of respondents indicated that education

Research in User Education 163

programs are being offered in any location that affords contact with users, such as halls, clinics, microcomputer labs across the campus, offices, laboratories, student unions, statewide meetings and conferences, or through electronic mail and the telephone. There appears to be a willingness to offer programs in any setting; however, equipment needs often preclude programs being taught in locations other than the library.

Financial Support

The number of users responding to questions relating to user education program support was only 27. Based on this small number of responses, it appears that the library budget is the main financial support for education programs. Eleven institutions (40.74 percent) indicated some but not more than 25 percent of their financial support comes from user fees. Only one institution indicated support from grants, and three institutions indicated support from contracts with specific user groups. Although the library budget supports the majority of education programs, 75 percent of the respondents reported that continuing financial support for user education is not clearly identifiable within the library's budget program and financial statements, nor are user education librarians clearly identifiable in the library's organizational chart (57.2 percent).

Program Offerings

Although most respondents reported the absence of a written profile of their community needs and no written statement of user education objectives, all respondents reported offering some user education programs. Respondents were asked to indicate both formal (75.9 percent) and informal (77.0 percent) education programs. Formal programs were described as classroom instruction of 30 minutes or more. Over three-fourths (75.9 percent) of the respondents offer formal and informal instruction on end-user database searching. Although Grateful MED might be subsumed under end-user database searching, the questionnaire was designed to elicit a separate response for instruction on Grateful MED. More libraries appear to offer informal instruction on Grateful MED (52.9 percent) than offer formal instruction (39.1 percent). The teaching of research methods appears to be offered by more libraries in the formal setting, whereas medical terminology is offered by more libraries in the informal setting. Analysis of the "other" category demonstrates that health sciences libraries are offering a variety of computer-related educational programs, such as the IBM Disc Operating System and a variety of microcomputer software packages for statistics, graphics, desktop publishing, and communication purposes.

FINDINGS AND CONCLUSIONS

There appears to be no relation between libraries having written profiles of their community's information needs and the number of types of programs they offer. The findings do indicate, however, that there is a difference in the number of types of program offerings and the existence of a written statement of user education objectives that serves as a guide for all user education programs in an institution ($t_{(84)} = -3.8995$; $p < .0002$). It appears that an institution which has a written statement of user education objectives will offer a greater variety of formal instructional programs than an institution which has no statement of objectives. The tests for significance also indicate that there is a strong relationship between the existence of a User Education Department and a greater variety of formal educational programs than when user education is left to subject specialists ($p < 0.0101$), a coordinator ($p < 0.0233$), a potpourri of staff ($p < 0.0048$), or the reference department ($p < 0.0022$).

Although health sciences libraries have come a long way, much work lies ahead for library directors to address the challenges proposed by the ALA Policy Statement demanding the same administrative funds and staffing support for user education as for more traditional library programs. This study shows all respondents (87) reported some level of user education, and all but four respondents offered formal education programs in 1988. It is clear, however, that user education does not share the same administrative and staffing support as do the more traditional library programs, nor have the 1977 ACRL *Guidelines* been realized in the majority of health sciences libraries. As the 1980s came to a close, the number of programs offered by health sciences libraries continued to grow to meet the technological changes in libraries, and user educators continued to search for funds and for the status they deserve.

Judging from the many comments of academic health sciences library directors, there is much interest in improving user education operations. Respondents indicated that additional education programs and some restructuring of positions will occur in the future to meet the growing demand for imparting information management skills. Others indicated that while there is a need for more user education programs, there is neither the personnel nor the budget to do more in this area.

This study does not go far enough. Studies similar to this one should examine the number of course offerings, the support staff who assist user education programs, and budgets as they relate to organizational structures. Through such studies we may better define and organize the management of user education.

REFERENCES

1. Griffin, Lloyd W., and Clarke, Jack A. "Orientation and Instruction of Graduate Students in the Use of University Library: A Survey." *College & Research Libraries* 133 (November 1972):471.

2. Runge, Elizabeth D. "Teaching the Use of the Library." *Bulletin of the Medical Library Association* 20 (July 1931):14-15.

3. "Policy Statement: Instruction in the Use of Libraries." *RSR* (Spring 1982):65.

4. "Guidelines for Bibliographic Instruction in Academic Libraries." *College and Research Libraries News* 38 (April 1977):92-93.

5. George, Mary W.; Hogan, Sharon A.; and Beaubien, Anne K. "Management Involvement in Library User Education: Inspiration, Toleration, or Participation." In: *Third International Conference on Library User Education.* University of Edinburgh July 19-22, 1983. Proceedings, Edited by Peter Fox and Ian Malloy, pp. 10-17. Edinburgh, Loughborough, 1983.

Chapter 17

CD-ROM MEDLINE Training:
A Survey of Medical School Libraries

Peggy W. Richwine
JoAnn H. Switzer

CD-ROM MEDLINE has created a whole new environment for
end-user searching in medical school libraries. Computerized access to medical journal literature at no cost to the user is attractive to
a great number of medical library users. Faculty or students, computer literates or unskilled typists, previous requesters of online
searches or persons completely unfamiliar with medical literature,
quickly become avid fans of CD-ROM MEDLINE. There are currently seven producers of CD-ROM MEDLINE products. The producers of CD-ROM MEDLINE indicate that the products are designed to be user-friendly. Observations have led librarians to
conclude that the CD-ROM user has little understanding of the
basics of searching. The resultant inference is that training in the
use of CD-ROM MEDLINE should be offered.

Medical librarians have traditionally provided training in how to
search the literature, whether the user is manually searching the
print indexes or running his own online searches, so that training for
end-user searching on CD-ROM MEDLINE is a natural extension
of reference services.

A survey was conducted in March 1989 to determine the extent
and nature of CD-ROM MEDLINE training. The survey focused on
the following aspects of this training:

This chapter was first published in *Medical Reference Services Quarterly*, Vol.
9(3), Fall 1990.

1. content of training;
2. the use of self-help aids;
3. scheduling and length of session;
4. evaluation of training.

This article discusses the importance of training the CD-ROM MEDLINE user, and analyzes the results of the survey.

LITERATURE REVIEW

End-user training has been available in some libraries since the 1970s and has become widespread in the 1980s. The impact of end-user training was noted by Wood: "the librarian's evolving role from search intermediary to consultant and educator . . . is a direct result of end-user searching."[1] Welborn, from a survey of all end-user training in medical school libraries, has identified the enhanced role in the academic community, increased self-esteem of the library staff, and the more positive view of librarians by clients as intangible rewards from the training of end users.[2]

The importance of the librarian in training the end user was noted as early as 1975 in the Olson study.[3] This study showed that non-librarian searchers have the best results when a librarian is involved in the training. Just as online end users need training, Miller has concluded that instruction is needed for CD-ROM users.[4] She noted that of the 500 search statements input by CD-ROM users, 37 percent produced no results because of errors. A total of 75 percent represented lost opportunities because of a lack of searching skills or a lack of knowledge of system-specific requirements. Miller wrote that user satisfaction was high. However, due to the nature of medical information and its intended use, CD-ROM users must be cautioned that the amount of data is vast and the necessary search strategies may be quite complex.

Plutchak's comments on the satisfied and inept user address the issue of what the goals of CD-ROM training are.[5] Setting goals for the training provides focus for the training content. Forms for evaluation of instruction may reflect the goals of the training and determine if these goals have been met.

THE SURVEY

The survey on CD-ROM MEDLINE training was sent to the United States libraries participating in the *Annual Statistics of Medical School Libraries in the United States and Canada (1977-1988).*[6] The survey questionnaire (see the Appendix) was designed as an information-gathering mechanism to provide a qualitative description of CD-ROM MEDLINE training and was not intended as a statistically valid instrument. Of the 127 questionnaires sent out, 81 libraries responded (a 64 percent response rate). Of these responses, 40 facilities had CD-ROM MEDLINE installations. These 40 responses were used for the tally on the utilization of self-help aids. Five of the facilities did not offer training for the CD-ROM user and were not used to tally the remaining questions.

RESULTS

A major part of any training is the written material that accompanies the verbal instruction. All but one of the sites that had CD-ROM installations had a written guide. Ten sites had vendor-produced guides only. For 12 sites an in-house produced guide was the only guide available to the user. Seventeen sites had both vendor and in-house produced guides. Many respondents with both types of guides found their in-house guides more useful than the vendor-produced guides. The majority of the 39 respondents considered them only somewhat useful, with less than one-fourth finding them very useful. Twelve respondents included a copy of their guide, which was designed as a quick reference tool by the user. All but one of these included operational instructions; nine had some reference to Medical Subject Headings and subheadings, limiting to English language, and the use of Boolean operators. Truncation and various ways to limit a search were included in half of the guides, while proximity searching was included in only one.

Another self-help tool that is available on some CD-ROMs is the ondisc tutorial. The survey question regarding these tutorials focused on how they are used. Of the 40 responses, 17 had systems that did not have a tutorial available. Among the other 23, 14 found

TABLE 17.1. Uses of CD Tutorials

USES OF TUTORIALS	NUMBER OF RESPONSES
Not at All	2
As a Refresher	3
Staff Unavailable	7
Major Form of Instruction	2
Introduction	14

the tutorial useful as an introduction. Three responses indicated the tutorial was the major form of instruction, while two others indicated the tutorial was not used at all. Some sites used the tutorial in multiple ways. Table 17.1 shows how the tutorial was used by the responding libraries.

One question concentrated on the scheduling of training sessions. Of the 34 responding, 28 (82 percent) offered individualized training, eight (24 percent) offered classes, and 22 (63 percent) had small group training. These sessions were done on demand in 47 percent of the libraries, by appointment in 32 percent of the libraries, and on a regularly scheduled basis in 38 percent. These percentages show that most facilities offered a variety of scheduling options.

Another aspect of scheduling is the length of the training session. Time intervals of five to ten minutes, 11 to 20 minutes, 21 to 40 minutes, and greater than 40 minutes were possible choices in this question. The breakdown of the group size by time interval is shown in Table 17.2. As can be seen from the Table, the larger groups had longer training sessions.

In order to determine if the initial training was the only training, the survey included a question on follow-up training. Of the 35 responses, 11 did not answer this question. Twenty-one responded that they offered follow-up training on an individualized, on-demand basis. Three sites offered advanced classes for follow-up training.

To determine the scope of the training, content of instruction was

TABLE 17.2. Length of Time of Initial CD Training

LENGTH OF TIME	INDIVIDUALIZED	SMALL GROUP	LARGE CLASSES
5-10 MIN	8	1	0
11-20 MIN	8	2	0
21-40 MIN	8	10	1
> 40 MIN	4	9	7
TOTAL	28	22	8

divided into ten categories with possible responses of "never," "sometimes," or "usually" for each category. The relationship to the print index, the need to divide a search into separate concepts, the use of Boolean operators, the role of Medical Subject Headings (MeSH) and subheadings, and various ways of limiting a search were included at least sometimes in the training at all locations. The use of MeSH trees and the explode command, use of proximity operators, and procedures for limiting to English language were never taught to the CD-ROM user in some facilities. The graph in Figure 17.1 shows the breakdown of these concepts and the frequency of their inclusion in the training.

According to the responses, evaluation of the training has been done at only five facilities. The respondents were asked what they had learned from the evaluation. "Users prefer hands-on training," "the librarian is the favorite form of instruction," "staff assistance is inadequate," and "the training was well received" were some of the comments. Two training evaluation forms were returned with the questionnaires. Both of these forms had an area for information about the trainee and an area for rating the content of the session and the presentation. Other questions focused on the parts of the training that were most useful, willingness to participate in advanced training, recommending the training to a peer, and whether the training met the stated objectives. Both forms reflected goals of user satisfaction but other goals were not clear from these forms.

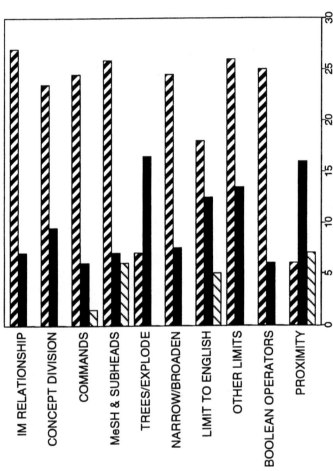

FIGURE 17.1. Content of CD Training

Legend: USUALLY, SOMETIMES, NEVER

SUMMARY

Based on the responses to this survey of medical school libraries, training of the CD-ROM MEDLINE user is being done in more than 85 percent of the libraries that subscribe to CD-ROM systems. Self-help tools such as quick reference guides and tutorials are used along with the instruction. Several training options are available at most libraries, with nearly one-fourth offering classes and more than three-fourths offering individualized training. Two-thirds of the training sessions are 20 minutes or more and 15 percent are ten minutes or less. Follow-up training is usually done on an individualized, on-demand basis with only three facilities offering classes beyond the initial training.

From the examination of the guides provided and the responses to the content question, the core of CD-ROM MEDLINE instruction includes its relationship to *Index Medicus*, dividing the search into concepts, use of Boolean operators, Medical Subject Headings and subheadings, and commands. Some of the ways of limiting a search and using search strategies to broaden or narrow a search are usually included. The use of MeSH trees, the explode command, and proximity operators are not generally a part of the initial training. Only five of the facilities that train CD-ROM MEDLINE users have evaluated the training.

CONCLUSION

The guides produced in-house show a tremendous duplication of effort. The Association of Academic Health Sciences Library Directors (AAHSLD) is sponsoring a project to develop "sharing kits" composed of training materials. Details on the availability of these kits can be found in the AAHSLD NEWS.[7]

Additional research is needed on goals and evaluation of the CD-ROM training and how this relates to the contents of the training. Investigation of variables such as prior computer or searching experience of CD-ROM trainees, length of time the library has had the CD-ROM installation, or location of CD-ROM workstations within the library might show a significant impact on the training that the CD-ROM MEDLINE user receives.

APPENDIX

INDIANA UNIVERSITY SCHOOL OF MEDICINE LIBRARY
COMPACT DISC MEDLINE QUESTIONNAIRE*

1. a. Do you have a manual or guide pages to assist the CD MEDLINE user?
    ____ yes   ____ no
    b. Is the guide ____ vendor produced   ____ created by you   ____ other.
    c. How useful do you consider the guide? ____ very   ____ somewhat   ____ slightly

2. a. Does your CD MEDLINE have a tutorial?   ____ yes   ____no
    b. Is the tutorial primarily used ____ as an introduction   ____ as the major form
    of instruction ____ when staff are not available to do training   ____ as a refresher
    ____ other (please specify)   _____.

3. Do you offer instruction for CD MEDLINE users? ____ yes   ____ no

4. In an average month how many initial trainings are done? _____
    How many followup trainings are done? _____

5. Which of these characterize your initial training? ____ class
    ____ individualized   ____ small groups   ____ regularly scheduled
    ____ by appointment   ____ on demand   ____ other

6. How long does your typical initial training last? ____ 5-10 minutes
    _____ 11-20 minutes   ____ 21-40 minutes   ____ > 40 minutes

7. Which of these characterize the follow-up training offered? ____ class
    ____ individualized   ____ small group   ____ regularly scheduled
    ____ by appointment   ____ on demand
    ____ other (please specify) _____

8. a. Have you done any written evaluation of your CD MEDLINE instruction?
    ____ yes   ____ no
    b. Use the space provided here to describe what you learned from the evaluation

    _____

    _____

9. Which of these aspects of searching MEDLINE does your initial CD training include?
    Please check the most appropriate column.

	never	sometimes	usually
a. discussion of relationship to *Index Medicus*	—	—	—
b. dividing a search into concepts	—	—	—
c. explanation of command structures	—	—	—
d. use of medical subject headings/subheadings	—	—	—
e. use of MESH trees and the explode command	—	—	—
f. strategies for narrowing/broadening a search	—	—	—
g. limiting the search to English	—	—	—
h. other ways of limiting the search	—	—	—
i. use of Boolean operators	—	—	—
j. use of proximity operators	—	—	—

* This is a portion of the original questionnaire

REFERENCES

1. Wood, M. Sandra. "End-User Searching: A Selected Annotated Bibliography." In: Wood, M. Sandra, Horak, Ellen B., and Snow, Bonnie, eds. *End-User Searching in the Health Sciences.* New York: The Haworth Press, 1986, pp. 213-274.

2. Welborn, Victoria, and Kuehn, Jennifer J. "End-User Programs in Medical School Libraries: A Survey." *Bulletin of the Medical Library Association* 16(April 1988):137-140.

3. Olson, Paul E. "Mechanization of Library Procedures in the Medium-Sized Medical Library: XV. A Study of the Interaction of Nonlibrarian Searchers with the MEDLINE Retrieval System." *Bulletin of the Medical Library Association,* 63(January 1975):35-39.

4. Miller, Naomi; Kirby, Martha; and Templeton, Etheldra. "MEDLINE on CD-ROM: End-User Searching in a Medical School Library." *Medical Reference Services Quarterly* 7(Fall 1988):1-13.

5. Plutchak, T. Scott. "On the Satisfied and Inept User." *Medical Reference Services Quarterly* 8(Spring 1989):45-48.

6. *Annual Statistics of Medical School Libraries in the United States and Canada 1987-88.* Houston, Texas: Houston Academy of Medicine-Texas Medical Center Library, 1989.

7. "Online Search Training by Academic Health Science Libraries." *AAHSLD News* 9(No. 1):1.

Chapter 18

An Analysis of Transaction Logs to Evaluate the Educational Needs of End Users

Janet L. Nelson

INTRODUCTION

In November of 1989, the University of Southern California (USC) introduced to its academic community a collection of online bibliographic databases known as USCInfo. The tapes of 13 databases were leased from various vendors and loaded on a mainframe computer at University Park Campus, thus permitting students, staff, and faculty to search free of charge from terminals in the numerous campus libraries and from their offices, laboratories, or homes, provided they had an access code, a personal computer, and either a modem or an Ethernet connection. Of prime importance to members of the Health Sciences Campus was that one of the databases consisted of the last ten years of MEDLINE records. The University offered four possible interfaces with which to search the system: BRS Native, BRS Colleague, BRS SearchMate, and a specially designed USCInfo interface. After careful consideration, the BRS Native and BRS Colleague interfaces were judged to be too difficult for the majority of end users, and the USCInfo interface, while user friendly, was not sophisticated enough to permit users to perform complicated searches. Therefore, the librarians of the

This chapter was first published in *Medical Reference Services Quarterly*, Vol. 11(4), Winter 1992.

Health Sciences Campus Library System decided to promote and support the BRS SearchMate interface.

At present, over 1,200 people at the Health Sciences Campus have received their own access codes. Last year over 60,000 logons were made and 15,000 hours of computing were used on USCInfo MEDLINE by Health Sciences Campus Library cardholders. Clearly end-user searching has gained widespread acceptance on the USC Health Sciences Campus and is here to stay.

END-USER EDUCATION

To support the system, the Information Services Department of USC Norris Medical Library has developed documentation explaining the features of the system, as well as the use of medical subject headings (MeSH), and offers two basic and one advanced class per month. The classes are held in the computer classroom which has 20 terminals, an instructor station, and a color projector for computer display. The classes consist of an hour lecture/demonstration, followed by a one-hour lab during which two instructors help users perform their own searches.

The present class structure and philosophy of end-user training evolved over the course of the first year. Initially, one two-hour class, covering everything from describing a bibliographic database to exploding a MeSH term, was offered. Although the class evaluations were consistently high, the instructors were dissatisfied with the outcome. Participants spent too much time on the basics and did not use MeSH during the lab session. It was then decided to split the course content into two sessions, MEDLINE Part I and MEDLINE Part II, and offer each class twice a month. Although the instructors were happy with the content of both courses, they noticed a tendency for participants to sign up for Part II immediately after Part I. Often those attending Part II had done no searching other than during the laboratory section of the Part I class. Too many of the questions asked in Part II related to basic skills covered in Part I. Once again the instructors decided that the participants were not focusing enough on the use of MeSH. It was felt that most people needed to have become familiar with the commands and to have had some experience searching on their own before the advantages of MeSH over Text Word searching became understandable. To discourage people from taking both classes within a few days of each other, it was decided to change the course names and the scheduling. Instead of Part I and Part II, the classes were renamed Basic MEDLINE and Advanced MEDLINE and the classes were scheduled farther apart. Basic is now offered twice a month and Advanced is taught once a month.

The Basic class covers the commands–how to log on, log off, print, limit, display, download, and perform crossfile searches. Additionally, how to construct a search strategy, the use of Boolean operators, the use of truncation, and the uses of field labels and positional operators are explained. Participants are shown how to refine their search strategy by picking up MeSH from the descriptor field of the record after an initial Text Word search.

In the Advanced class, it is assumed that the searcher has conquered the basic mechanics and commands of the system and is ready to concentrate on the use of the MeSH vocabulary. Topics covered include major descriptors, subheadings, exploding, exploding a major descriptor, pre-explodes, and subheading pre-explodes. Copies of *Medical Subject Headings–Annotated Alphabetic List*, *Medical Subject Headings–Tree Structures*, and *Permuted Medical Subject Headings* are available in the classroom and time is spent examining them. Information on purchasing these books from the National Library of Medicine is provided.

In addition to these classes, USCInfo MEDLINE training has become a required part of the curriculum for all first-year medical students and third-year pharmacy students. Also, special classes for various groups are scheduled upon request. For example, this year instruction was offered to 13 groups, including premed students, physicians' assistants, medical education fellows, occupational therapists, and residents and interns in several departments. Also, an individual who because of time constraints either cannot attend a regularly scheduled class or has an immediate need may make an appointment with an instructor for a private tutorial. Over 600 people took one of the classes last year. In all of these classes, the use of MeSH to obtain optimal results was advocated.

Additionally, informal training is provided as time permits at three stations near the reference desk. Although numerous opportunities exist for users to obtain formal instruction, some users prefer to train themselves with or *without* reading the documentation. A one-page handout that would enable a first-time user to perform a simple subject or author search was created to assist those who do not have the patience to read the documentation. Even this short self-help aid contains the caveat, "For best search results, use medical subject headings."

TRANSACTION LOGS

In an attempt to evaluate how end users are searching and to assess their instructional needs, one week of transaction logs were examined. Since the week was December 10-16, 1991, pharmacy, first- and second-year medical students, and students enrolled in other health-sciences-related programs would not be heavily represented in this group because they had either started Christmas break or were taking final examinations. Thus, the primary focus was on the searching behaviors of faculty, staff, and third- and fourth-year medical students–those individuals who had not been required to take training on the system, but may have elected to do so.

The transaction logs included both those searching in the library and those searching from remote terminals. After excluding the searches done by librarians during that week and the searches done in databases other than MEDLINE, 643 searches were left. As shown in Figure 18.1, 73 percent of the searches were subject searches (subject/journal title and subject/address searches were included here), 25.5 percent were author searches (author/subject and author/ address searches were included in this category), and 1.5 percent were classified as "other" searches (nine address searches, one failed journal title search).

These were re-input into the system by the reference staff and divided into three categories: those producing zero retrieval, those producing marginal results, and those that were judged as successful. Yasar Tonta pointed out that while "transaction monitoring is the most appropriate technique to study search failures when the cause(s) of search failures are obvious (e.g., zero retrieval due to misspelling or collection failures) . . . partial failures can best be

FIGURE 18.1. Types of Searches

	NUMBER	PERCENT
SUBJECT	468	73.0%
AUTHOR	165	25.5%
OTHER	10	1.5%
	(N = 643)	

studied with the help of the user."[1] Nevertheless, for the purpose of this study, some measure of marginal success (i.e., partial failure), however imperfect, needed to be established by the evaluator without the help of the user. When examining transaction logs, one comes across searches with positive retrievals that are so obviously flawed that a conscientious database searcher cannot lump them in with the successful searches.

ANALYSIS

Figure 18.2 shows that 84 percent of the searches were judged to be successful; 8 percent produced marginal results; and 8 percent provided zero retrieval. The success rate was fairly high when compared to similar studies.[2-4] Clearly, most people were able to overcome difficulties with the mechanics of the system either through instruction, documentation, or sheer perseverance in a "trial and error" approach, and most searches obtained some results.

The author searches were fairly straightforward. Eighty-one percent were successful, 4 percent were marginal, and 15 percent had zero results. The reasons for zero or marginal retrievals were: (1) the name was not in the database; (2) the proper author format was not used; or (3) the author was searched only by a common last name, thus producing too large a retrieval. Of the successful searches, 72 percent were entered in the proper format; 28 percent were not, but,

FIGURE 18.2. Success Rates for Searches

	SUCCESS	MARGINAL	ZERO RESULTS
TOTAL	84% (n = 538)	8% (n = 53)	8% (n = 52)
SUBJECT	85% (n = 397)	10% (n = 45)	5% (n = 26)
AUTHOR	81% (n = 134)	4% (n = 7)	15% (n = 24)
OTHER	70% (n = 7)	1% (n = 1)	20% (n = 2)
	(n = 643)		

nonetheless, gave positive results. The reasons that author searches which were not in proper format succeeded were: (1) the author did not have a common last name, (2) two or more authors' last names were combined, or (3) the author's last name was combined with a keyword in the title or abstract.

Of the subject searches, 85 percent were judged successful; 10 percent were marginal; and 5 percent produced zero retrieval. Reasons for a subject search being judged a marginal success include:

1. retrieving too many results, causing one to logoff immediately without printing or displaying;
2. using a stopword that significantly throws off retrieval;
3. obtaining a few valid results, but missing the majority due to faulty technique or poor vocabulary;
4. obtaining results all of which were invalid.

Examples include a searcher who retrieved 300 records and logged off immediately without displaying or printing; a searcher who input "diagnosis of arthritis" and retrieved only records containing the words arthritis and diagnosis coupled with the MeSH "activities-of-daily-living"; a searcher who used the term "tumours" and retrieved only British articles; and a searcher who used the word "English" (instead of limiting to English) and obtained only foreign language articles having English abstracts. These searches were all deemed to have obtained marginal results.

Subject searches were not evaluated as to whether or not a trained database searcher could produce better results; one would certainly expect a professional searcher to do a better job. Nor were Text Word searches evaluated as to whether they could be improved upon by using MeSH; the indexers at the National Library of Medicine would probably hope that in most cases this would prove true. The primary goal in providing documentation and training for USC-Info MEDLINE is to enable end users to find information that will help them make informed decisions. It is not expected that the majority of users will develop the same high level of skill that is expected of a medical librarian.

When the 397 successful subject searches were further analyzed to determine the levels of skill of the searchers, it was discovered that 21 percent (n = 114) of the successful searches demonstrated no skill at all, other than typing words together on one line. Also, as shown in Figure 18.3, the majority of the searches did not use such helpful techniques as limiting to language, truncating, combining synonyms with ORs or using positional operators such as ADJ. Despite making training and documentation readily available, only 20 percent used MeSH in at least one search statement; the other 80 percent relied solely on Text Words. This result was remarkably similar to results found by Horres, who stated "more than 20 percent of the searches for topical material in MELVYL MEDLINE contained keywords rather than controlled vocabulary headings."[5]

DISCUSSION

More people at the Health Sciences Campus are receiving more information than ever before. Prior to making end-user searching available, the mediated search load never approached 538 searches a week, i.e., the number of successful searches done during the week of this study. The maximum was on the average of 30 a week, and it is highly unlikely that manual searching would account for the extra 508 successful searches. Therefore, people are finding information that in the past they would have done without.

However, while some searchers are doing sophisticated searching using advanced techniques, most are not. The need to inform the end user that he may be, in fact most probably is, missing important

FIGURE 18.3. Skills Used in Successful Subject Searching

SKILL	NUMBER	PERCENT
One or more skills used	283	79%
Combines sets	194	49%
Limits	82	21%
Uses MeSH	80	20%
MeSH/subheading combination	30	8%
MeSH/attached subheading	18	5%
MeSH/floating or exploded subheading	12	3%
Use of .de. for descriptor	14	3.5%
Use of .mj. for major descriptor	14	3.5%
Explodes	9	2.5 %
Positional operators	49	12%
Review articles	39	9%
ORs	31	8%
Parenthesis (nested terms)	23	6%
Age groups	19	5%
Keyword in title	21	5%
Crossfiles	19	5%
Truncation	13	3%
Not	12	3%
Keyword in abstract	10	2.5%

(n = 397)

FIGURE 18.4. Further Observations Concerning Subject Searches

Observation	NUMBER	PERCENT
Use of stopwords	13	3%
Fails to use crossfile	58	14.5%
Poor choice of Text Word	54	14%
Searches backfile also	77	19.5%
Uses subheadings as Text Words	28	7%
Picks up MeSH from record	14	3.5%
Average number of search statements per search	7.3	
(n = 397)		

information is ever present. End users should be aware that mediated searches in most instances will provide more complete results, and they should also be able to recognize those situations in which end-user searches are inappropriate, e.g., critical patient care.

Better methods to encourage end users to use MeSH to improve their results need to be developed. Despite our adopted roles as "MeSH missionaries," 80 percent of the searchers are still unconverted. Systems such as Grateful Med or PaperChase, which encourage the use of medical subject headings, subheadings, and explodes, may provide the user with more satisfactory results. Consideration should be given to developing an interface for a locally mounted MEDLINE database that promotes the use of MeSH.

If user preference is for Text Word searching, end users should be taught to use Text Words more effectively. Because of the low usage of truncation (3 percent), OR's (9 percent), and positional operators (12 percent), and the relatively high percentage of poor selection of Text Words (14 percent), as shown in Figures 18.3 and 18.4, there is an obvious immediate need for users to improve Text Word searching skills.

Efforts need to be made to give those searching the system further instruction. The searcher with experience is more apt to grasp some of the finer points of using MeSH and to appreciate some of the underutilized features of the system, e.g., crossfile searching, now that he has a firm foundation of the basic mechanics.

CONCLUSION

In short, although end users are currently performing thousands of searches each year at the USC Health Sciences Campus, librarians need to develop ways to encourage users to become more effective and more sophisticated searchers. Possible ways to meet this challenge include sponsoring a USCInfo MEDLINE users group, offering "brown bag" lunch demonstrations on various topics such as "Ten Ways to Improve Your MEDLINE Retrievals," writing additional documentation to steer users away from making the most common errors, and offering refresher classes to those who want to refine their skills. Also, a user survey which asks very specific questions such as "Do you use ADJ to search a phrase?" could prove helpful. Such a survey would not only provide valuable information, but also would heighten the users' awareness of the availability of the many underutilized features of the system. The librarians at the Norris Medical Library are committed to teaching end users to search MEDLINE more effectively and are willing to devote the necessary time and energy required to explore new methods to promote better end-user searches.

REFERENCES

1. Tonta, Y. "Analysis of Search Failures in Document Retrieval Systems: A Review." *Public-Access Computer Systems Review* 3 (no. 1, 1992):4-53.

2. Miller, N.; Kirby, M.; and Templeton, E. "MEDLINE on CD-ROM: End User Searching in a Medical School Library." *Medical Reference Services Quarterly* 7 (Fall 1988):1-13.

3. Cahan, M. A. "Grateful MED: A Tool for Studying Searching Behavior." *Medical Reference Services Quarterly* 8 (Winter 1989):61-79.

4. Walker, C. J.; McKibbon, K. A.; Haynes, R. B.; and Ramsden, M. F. "Problems Encountered by Clinical End Users of MEDLINE and Grateful Med." *Bull. Med. Libr. Assoc* 79 (January 1991):67-69.

5. Horres, M. M.; Starr, S. S.; and Renford, B. L. "MELVYL MEDLINE: A Library Services Perspective." *Bull. Med. Lib. Assoc.* 79 (July 1991):309-320.

PART IV

INFORMATION MANAGEMENT EDUCATION AND COMPUTER LITERACY PROGRAMS

Chapter 19

New Roles for the Medical Librarian in an Information Management Environment

Diane G. Schwartz

INTRODUCTION

Traditionally, the library has been the medical center's primary information handling unit. Over the course of the next 20 years libraries will be retooled to function as the hub of the medical center's information network. This will result in expanded responsibilities for the librarian, including managing the quality of information flowing through the network, and developing filtering techniques that organize information so that it responds to problem-solving and instructional needs.

Automation has helped establish librarians as experts in the design of new hardware and software products and the development of new instructional programs. In assuming these new roles, librarians have learned to successfully market their products and services.[1] None of these skills are new to librarians; rather, they have taken on a new dimension, and as Lancaster has said, they have established the librarian's role as a communicator.[2]

As we progress toward an automated information environment,

This chapter is an adaptation of a paper presented at the Midwest Chapter/Medical Library Association Meeting, October 25-27, 1984, Cedar Rapids, IA, entitled, "The Matheson Report and Beyond–Implications for Library Use Instruction and Information Management Education." This chapter was first published in *Medical Reference Services Quarterly*, Vol. 6(4), Winter 1987.

librarians will be seeking answers to several questions: (1) How do we utilize developing technologies to organize information so that we can make necessary decisions with ease? (2) How do we educate library users to function effectively in this rapidly changing, technologically complex environment? (3) How will the new environment change the responsibilities of the medical librarian?

The goal of this chapter is to describe the expanded roles awaiting medical librarians, the technological changes likely to occur in health sciences libraries, the new services librarians will offer, and the dilemmas librarians may experience as a result of these changes. The period of change will be divided into the 13 years of 1988-2000, and the turn of the century and beyond.

EXPANDED ROLES FOR LIBRARIANS: 1988-2000

The technological changes occurring from 1988 to 2000 will expand and refine existing functions and services. For example, the library will have an online catalog and physicians will either own a microcomputer or have access to file space in the medical center's mainframe computer. In many communities both practicing physicians and medical center staff will, through local area networks, be able to gain access to the medical center's mainframe computer to transfer information from a variety of databases to their own files.[3]

In this environment, librarians will teach courses on the development of personal information filing systems, offer advice on the selection of software, teach clients to access the library's online catalog, and provide instruction in conducting database searches using end-user search systems. Librarians will teach online composition, editing and refereeing of online journal articles, and the construction of specialized knowledge bases. Finally librarians will create computer-assisted instruction programs to teach problem-solving skills.[4]

Technology will alter a librarian's typical work day. Those database searches still run by librarians will be more complex and more time-consuming. Professional librarians will spend fewer hours at the reference desk; instead, they will be on duty at electronic work stations, interacting with users via electronic mail and network linkages.[3]

EXPANDED ROLES FOR LIBRARIANS:
2000 AND BEYOND

By the turn of the twenty-first century word processing systems will have voice recognition and voice input capabilities. Most current library materials will be stored on videodiscs; older materials will be kept in centralized regional facilities with copies transmitted via telefacsimile as needed. Some journals will remain in print while others will be available in an electronic mode only. Journal article usage will be recorded online by users and will serve as a measure of quality.[3] Specialized knowledge bases will be available in most disciplines; they will serve as online encyclopedias that are updated regularly. Knowledge bases in the clinical disciplines will be linked to research knowledge bases for rapid dissemination of the most recent findings. The linkage will occur through the medical center's local area network.[3]

Librarians may work in decentralized information units based on their subject knowledge and expertise. Their responsibilities will mirror the duties performed today by clinical medical librarians, but they will rely more heavily on electronic network and interface capabilities. The title "Librarian" may be replaced by the title "Information Specialist." Working under any title, these professionals will be creators of information products and teachers. They will work with physicians to create knowledge bases that will replace traditional textbooks, and they will design interpretive information products that provide commentaries on a single topic from a wide range of sources and from divergent points of view.[3] These professionals will teach active informed learning techniques that stress "learning how to learn" in a qualitative sense, while providing the foundation for helping physicians to identify their own learning needs. Emphasis will be on teaching the use of the computer as an extended memory device, replacing the rote acquisition of facts with the broad study of decision processes and strategies.[5] Librarians will develop an intimate familiarity with the medical center's information network and teach the staff to exploit the system to its fullest potential.

In addition to their instructional duties, Information Specialists will function as information analyzers, synthesizing results from a variety of sources and presenting evaluated mini reviews of the literature. An answer to a question is provided rather than a bibliography.[2]

As we proceed into the twenty-first century, microcomputers will become sophisticated workstations that enable clinicians, researchers, and librarians to receive, compose, and search for text. The information sought may be found in either public domain or commercial databases, or in knowledge bases created by colleagues working in closely related fields, but separated geographically.[6]

Information Specialists will spend more of their time performing information transfer functions, and teaching others these skills. As a result of changed commitments, those traditional reference services that are offered will be handled increasingly by paraprofessionals. The library will be less a repository of books and journals than a management system for a variety of computer-stored files. As the concept of the Information Specialist takes root, and as staff improve their information management skills, there will be a greater effort to match the skills of these professionals with the specialized needs of physicians and researchers.[3] Increasingly, Information Specialists will need training in the disciplines they serve so that they will be able to evaluate data, relate the results to the existing knowledge base, and bring an interdisciplinary perspective to their teaching and information transfer responsibilities.

DILEMMAS LIBRARIANS MAY EXPERIENCE

As the computer becomes more fully integrated into library operations and accepted by staff, several questions will emerge. For example, what will be the relationship of the library to the computing center? Will there be a collegial relationship, or will one unit report to the other? At present there seems to be no clear answer to either question.

The issue of bibliographic access and control will require a good deal of time to sort out, and will probably not be resolved until after the turn of the century. Changed book and journal selection responsibilities, i.e., selecting what to access to satisfy a known need, rather than what to purchase, will require time and retraining to accomplish. Finally, in "the very near future, one of the librarian's main jobs will be . . . discarding inappropriate" information.[7]

EPILOGUE

While the dilemmas are serious, to date librarians have made significant progress in the move to create an automated, electronic library. Some of the real accomplishments that have taken place in providing electronic access to information include:

- The knowledge base research program of the Lister Hill Center at the National Library of Medicine, resulting in the development of the Hepatitis Knowledge Base.[8]
- The Integrated Library System developed by the National Library of Medicine and made available in 1980.
- PaperChase, a computer program that enables physicians to search the medical literature and retrieve materials actually available in their institution's medical library.[9]
- Simultaneous remote search, first reported by librarians and physicians at the Tucson, Arizona Medical Center. It enables physicians and librarians to work together to formulate and conduct a search using an interactive telecommunications system despite the fact that they are separated geographically.[10]
- User-friendly search systems such as BRS/Colleague, DIALOG's Knowledge Index and Medis.
- Integrated Academic Information Management Systems (IAIMS).[11]

CONCLUSION

To date considerable progress has been made in understanding what the effect of technology will be on medical libraries. To achieve the changes described above, libraries must be retooled to serve as information transfer networks, and they must become the medical center's resource for academic information management services. Librarians must begin to develop formalized instructional programs that will link individuals to information and to systems that provide those individuals with personal memory extenders and lifelong learning supports. As librarians become Information Specialists/Managers they must recognize that their "first mission . . . is to integrate . . . internal information resources–both physical and intellectual–to make them efficient and effective in supporting the work of the organization." Second, they must "filter the external knowledge base in order to bring in only that which is relevant and useful."[12] In the process, librarians will develop the skills needed to function as:

- Interpreters of interdisciplinary information
- Information analyzers
- Exploiters of electronic information sources
- Interpreters of information products.

Finally, librarians must change their image. They must recognize their areas of expertise and they must begin now to promote that expertise. If they do not, someone else will come along and claim information management as their domain.

REFERENCES

1. Bloom, P.N. "Effective Marketing for Professional Services." *Harv Bus Rev* 620 (Sept.-Oct. 1984):102-110.
2. Lancaster, W.F. "Future Librarianship: Preparing for an Unconventional Career." *Wilson Lib Bul* 57 (May 1983):747-753.
3. Matheson, N.W., and Cooper, J.A.D. "Academic Information in the Academic Health Science Center: Roles for the Library in Information Management." *J Med Educ* 57 Part 2 (October 1982).
4. Lancaster, W.F.; Drasgow, L.; and Marks, E. *Impact of a Paperless Society on the Research Library of the Future; A Report to the National Science Foundation.* Urbana, IL: University of Illinois, 1980.
5. "Evaluation of Medical Information Science in Medical Education." *J Med Educ* 61 (June 1986):487-543.
6. Battin, P. "The Electronic Library–A Vision for the Future." *EDUCOM Bull* 19(Summer 1984):12-17, 34.

7. Atkinson, N.C. "Who Will Run and Use Libraries?" *Libr J* 109(Oct. 15, 1984):1905-1907.

8. Bernstein, L.M.; Siegel, E.R.; and Goldstein, C.M. "The Hepatitis Knowledge Base; A Prototype Information Transfer System." *Ann Intern Med* 93 Part 2 (July 1980):165-222.

9. Horowitz, G.L., and Bleich, H.L. "PaperChase: A Computer Program to Search the Medical Literature." *New Engl J Med* 305(Oct. 15, 1981):924-930.

10. Graham, D.L.; King, C.; and Whitney, P.J. "Simultaneous Remote Search; On-line Bibliographic Library Services for Practicing Physicians." *JAMA* 246(Sept. 4, 1981):1115-1116.

11. "Symposium on Academic Information in the Academic Health Sciences Center: Roles for the Library in Information Management." *Bull Med Libr Assoc* 71(Oct. 1983):404-434.

12. Daniel, E.N. "Educating the Academic Librarian for a New Role as Information Resources Manager." *J Acad Libr* 11(Jan. 1986):360-364.

Chapter 20

Teaching Computer Literacy:
Helping Patrons to Help Themselves

Elizabeth H. Wood

If this chapter were to be indexed, it would probably be assigned the terms LIBRARIES, MEDICAL; LIBRARY SERVICES; EDU–CATION, MEDICAL; and MICROCOMPUTERS. While these are indeed the subjects involved, a further aspect of this discussion is a new heading that could be coined: LIBRARIAN-PATRON RELA-TIONS. Developments in user education that are the result of technological advances have changed and continue to change the relations between librarian and user.[1] This chapter is both a description of the programs and services offered at the University of Southern California (USC) Norris Medical Library, hereinafter referred to as "Norris," as well as a discussion of their effect in the local context and the implications for the wider context of medical librarianship. The focus here is the adaptation of the librarian's traditional role to meet another technological change, and the need for an integrated approach to a computer literary program.

"LITERACY"

The expression "computer literacy" is interesting; there is nothing new in the role of the librarian as the teacher of literacy. There was a time in the Middle Ages when librarians not only collected

This chapter is based on a presentation of the same title at the 87th Annual Meeting of the Medical Library Association, Portland, OR, May 1987. This chapter was first published in *Medical Reference Services Quarterly*, Vol. 7(3), 1988.

and kept the books but were among the few people who could *read* them. Lord Kenneth Clark, in his book, *Civilisation,* comments on Charlemagne's efforts in this area:

> . . . it is a great convenience to be able to read and write.
>
> For over five hundred years this achievement was rare in Western Europe. It is a shock to realise that during all this time practically no lay person, from kings and emperors downwards, could read or write. Charlemagne learnt to read, but he never could write. He had wax tablets beside his bed to practise on, but said he couldn't get the hang of it.[2]

There is such a tempting parallel in online information systems. Until only a few years ago, users depended upon librarians to learn the command languages of database searching and perform the searches. Many librarians are now teaching those very skills to users. Literacy gives access to information. Bibliographic instruction guides the literate user in finding the information. Computer literacy further enhances the process. As pointed out by Francesca Allegri, computerization has merely drawn attention to the bibliographic instruction that many librarians have always done.[3] Allegri further points out that libraries with small budgets which cannot afford the necessary hardware and software should not be assumed to lack teaching skills or opportunities. Much of the reference work is teaching patrons to use information sources to best advantage, whether printed or online.

COMPUTER LITERACY FOR LIBRARIANS

Library education has absorbed technological advances as they have appeared. At one point in history, penmanship was a requisite of library education.[4] Later in time, librarians who could not use a typewriter were at a disadvantage. Training in the use of computerized sources is now standard. At Norris, librarians who are not already familiar with personal computers are given systematic training in the use of a disk operating system, word processors, telecommunications packages, and a number of user-friendly programs that are used for workshops and demonstrations as well for their own searching. Little distinction is made between the need to understand the organization of printed indexes and the principles involved in the compilation of computerized files.

In a large library it is important that all the librarians be aware of one another's skills and the programs being used; this enables staff to help one another in learning new programs or systems and avoids duplication in acquiring software and manuals. Computers and programs are found in every department of the Norris library; there is a local area network and electronic mail service available within the library and across the campus. Since the coordination of computer activities cuts across the traditional divisions of Technical and Public Services and Learning Resources, a new position was created, called "Computer Services Librarian." The accumulated knowledge and experience of all the librarians are used to maintain a computer literacy teaching program that benefits both librarians and users. While none of the elements of the Norris program are unique,[5-6] the activities and facilities described below are extensive, and the experiences and conclusions of Norris staff may help others who are considering developing a similar program.

PREPARATION FOR TEACHING COMPUTER LITERACY

Assuming that librarians have acquired the necessary skills, there are several major considerations in preparing to teach computer literacy. They include: costs of hardware, software, and online connect time; provision of a teaching environment; staff time for class preparation and teaching; and advertising the program.

Costs

Many libraries are now charging fees for teaching computer skills or for using computer facilities within the library. The high cost of computer hardware and software, to which may be added the need for additional electrical outlets, telephone lines, and special furniture, may force a library to charge fees on a cost-recovery basis. Other libraries may have to justify the acquisition of computer equipment by offering evidence in advance that these costs can be recovered. This can mean they are in the business of selling their services.[7-9] Both hardware and software producers may provide free material for educational purposes. In the case of software, Norris has had considerable success in obtaining demonstration copies and even full programs from producers who are aware that the library is providing them with free publicity by demonstrating their programs. Many online database vendors are similarly willing to provide free connect time and passwords.

Space

As in the Norris experience, classes of up to a dozen participants can be taught in a room with only 600 square feet, using a portable PC, floppy disks, and a 25-inch monitor. The room may not need to be in the library itself. When the classes become popular, space may be offered by other departments or the library may request special funding to build a computer teaching facility.

Advertising

Even if classes are offered free of charge, librarians may need to convince users that they need to learn these new skills. To accomplish this they may publish newsletters, organize user groups, and invite salespeople from database vendors or software producers to give presentations to both librarians and patrons.

It may not be possible to predict the popularity or extent of end-user programs. The program may grow gradually, therefore, and the need for tighter organization may only become apparent as the demand increases. Initially, one librarian may devise a workshop outline, write some handout notes, design a flyer, and arrange for the use of a room and some kind of display equipment. The extensive program and facilities at Norris, described below, were not part of an original master plan. As more librarians began teaching workshops, a coordinator was designated, and flyers were combined into one overall listing. Instead of choosing a time and place to fit a particular librarian's work schedule, the workshops had to be planned together, well in advance, ensuring that equipment and space would be available, and that programs did not conflict. The four computer user groups developed along similar lines. At first there was only one. By the time the third group began to hold regular meetings, patrons complained that it was difficult to attend more than one in a week. These groups also had to be centrally controlled and coordinated. Coordination can be a major task; at Norris, it has become a major part of some librarians' jobs to organize and plan for activities that did not exist only a few years ago. An extensive program in teaching computer literacy is certainly not something that libraries can undertake overnight, or without the resources and staffing to provide the necessary training and supervision.

What effect do all these activities have on the relationship between librarian and patron? How does this change the role of the librarian, on a personal level, among colleagues, and among users? What is the effect of teaching users to help themselves to sources of information that were once available only through the intermediary of the librarian? These questions will be addressed as the programs and activities at Norris are described.

THE NORRIS COMPUTER ACTIVITIES

As the description of the *what, where, when,* and *how* of the Norris Library programs unfolds, various perspectives will be examined, leading to the conclusion that the library as a place of learning and the librarian as an information professional must inevitably derive new energy from these technological developments. Increased computer literacy of librarians enables them to be teachers and consultants for users who need to take advantage of automated access to information.

The computer activities of the Information Services Division of the Norris Medical Library, USC Health Sciences Library System, fall into four major categories. These are: workshops on aspects of database management and bibliographic database searching, provision of a microcomputer laboratory and special staff to help users with hardware and software, formation of computer user groups, and provision and maintenance of a Health Sciences Campus electronic bulletin board.

INFORMATION MANAGEMENT WORKSHOPS

Workshops are the most direct route by which the library is teaching computer literacy. At Norris there is a series of six workshops designed to help health professionals gain access to medical and pharmaceutical information. The emphasis is on the use of MEDLINE, the online index to the biomedical literature produced by the National Library of Medicine (NLM). The workshops are:

- USING YOUR PC TO SEARCH ONLINE DATABASES
- MeSH AND TEXTWORD SEARCHING
- SEARCHING MEDLINE USING NLM'S COMMAND LANGUAGE
- FRONTEND AND GATEWAY SOFTWARE
- REPRINT FILE MANAGEMENT
- DOWNLOADING AND CITATION MANAGEMENT

USING YOUR PC and FRONTEND SOFTWARE overlap somewhat but the emphases are different; one is more concerned with telecommunications and the other with search-aid software. Many participants in the PC class are already using their machines for word processing or other office applications and want to learn what other uses are possible.

The MeSH class can be used as an introduction to SEARCHING MEDLINE, or after that class, for students who want to become more sophisticated. The SEARCHING MEDLINE class (which used to be the NLM presentation entitled "The Basics of Searching MEDLINE") is still very popular even though it is no longer required for obtaining an NLM password. It is offered about once a month, sometimes as one eight-hour class, and sometimes in two four-hour sessions. The other seminars are from three to four hours in length and are deliberately offered at different times–both during the day and on evenings and weekends.

FRONTEND AND GATEWAY SOFTWARE usually concentrates on one program such as Grateful MED, Pro-Search, Paper-Chase, or Med-Base. One of the most recent developments in what may be called search-aid software is the availability of databases on CD-ROM. Free MEDLINE searching on CD-ROM disks is offered at Norris and included in the workshop. This has attracted some users, not because they are particularly interested in MEDLINE, but because they want to see the CD and its player.

The REPRINT seminar has two forms. One is strictly for manual indexing systems and discusses classifying and physically filing a reprint collection, and the other demonstrates a number of software packages indicating the good and bad points of each and giving an overview of what is available on the market.

DOWNLOADING follows logically from a number of the others; it takes the approach of, "So now you know how to search, but what can you do with all those lists of references?" It includes, as do most of the others, demonstrations of programs that are representative of the market. These workshops are taught in the microcomputer classroom (which will be described later) where each participant can have hands-on practice.

The workshops are publicized widely on the campus to faculty, students, and staff. The majority of the participants have been faculty; staff members, particularly at the administrative assistant level, have been the next largest group. Medical students have little free time to devote to optional classes or workshops. Good rapport has been generated between faculty and librarians. Attendees have come back to the library with their searching experiences, to tell librarians about software programs they have purchased as a result of the demonstrations, to ask questions and to share discoveries. Librarians have been invited to give versions of the seminars to community hospitals or be guest lecturers to classes in other schools at the university. The workshops on database searching have not diminished the library's search load; indeed, the effect has been greater visibility and awareness of searching. While many users are doing their own searching, others are requesting searches to be done more frequently. The number of searches performed by librarians has increased more than 30 percent in the past year alone. A less desirable result has been desperate telephone calls from frustrated searchers who are "stuck" in the middle of a search and wondering what to do next! Similarly, librarians who have demonstrated software are called upon to help users who have purchased it and to advise on ways to use it to best advantage.

The effects of this teaching program on reference librarians have been the accumulation of skills in using microcomputers, contact with users who may not otherwise use the library, awareness of faculty and staff research projects and subject areas, enhanced participation in local and national library organizations, and personal relationships with users that have improved LIBRARIAN-PA-TRON RELATIONS.

MICROCOMPUTER FACILITIES

Norris has two microcomputer rooms: a laboratory with 15 IBM machines and six Macintoshs, and a classroom with 20 IBMs and a teacher's station. The laboratory is open at all times and is staffed during daytime and evening hours and on Saturdays by a computer expert. The classroom, on the other hand, is available only to faculty (and librarians) and must be reserved for teaching purposes. It contains a blackboard, large screen and color projector for computer display, and a regular overhead projector. Additional computers, a laser disk reader, two CD-ROM players, and two end-user search stations are available in the Learning Resources Center. Over 200 software programs are available for check-out and use within the library; many popular programs are loaded onto hard disks. Students, staff, and faculty are encouraged to learn word processing, spreadsheets, statistical analysis, database management, authoring languages, and interactive instruction. A number of faculty have devised their own computer-assisted teaching programs. This computer facility has resulted in librarian and faculty contact that may not otherwise have taken place. At times, librarians' knowledge of which buttons to press next has been pushed to the limits, forcing them to improve their own skills. The Computer Services Librarian has organized classes to train the Norris librarians, to learn from one another's experiences and to improve everyone's conceptual framework. An in-house database has been established to identify which library divisions have acquired manuals, tutorials, and copies of articles that can be loaned to others. The effect of providing the latest in technology is that professionals have to extend their areas of expertise. A further unforeseen result is that librarians are invited to establish computer workstations and online searching equipment in offices and laboratories.

COMPUTER USER GROUPS

There are four computer user groups that meet regularly for noontime, brown-bag sessions:

- Educational Applications Microcomputer User Group
- Office Applications Microcomputer User Group
- Scientific Computer Applications User Group
- Health Sciences Campus Online User Group

The groups vary in type of presentation, audience, and amount of participation on the part of the librarian in charge of each group.[10] The educational applications group is usually run by faculty members, showing each other their teaching or testing techniques using computers. The office applications group often features presentations by library staff and discusses word processing, spreadsheets, printers, and the like. The scientific applications group features outside speakers, invited by the librarian, who talk about programs written for minis or mainframes, number crunchers, artificial intelligence, etc. The librarian sometimes just sits back and listens. The online user group (composed largely of past students from the seminars) discusses searching problems and learns from others' experiences. From time to time a topic of general interest is presented at a combined meeting of all four groups. Such topics have included presentations by a central university authority responsible for the campus-wide installation of a new voice and data telephone system, and a demonstration by a major computer manufacturer of the latest significant new product line. As a whole, these meetings bring people into the library who would perhaps not otherwise have come and provide exposure for librarians in contexts other than the reference desk or the classroom. Norris librarians have become more aware of the specific interests and research areas of the faculty and staff and have established many personal contacts.

ELECTRONIC BULLETIN BOARD

The electronic bulletin board provides a service for the Health Sciences campus. The library posts routine messages about hours, loan policies, calendars of workshops and meetings, and the text of newsletters, new acquisitions lists, and flyers. There is also a menu of files that can be downloaded, such as fellowships that are available and research being conducted at the university. Whole departments may apply for passwords that are on various levels, enabling them to leave messages open to all, or only to particular departments or individuals. During the installation of the bulletin board the librarian who acts as "SYSOP" (or "system operator") of the board talked to faculty members and students about the hardware and software the library was considering as well as the market for this type of program. The board has a "Chat" option: when a user types the letter "C" a bell chimes in the office enabling the SYSOP to break in to chat online with the user. In this way librarians have "conversed" digitally with faculty and staff they have never met. The effect, once more, is contact for the library with new users–groups of people who may not otherwise be library users. The bulletin board, unlike the workshops and user groups, has attracted students as well as faculty and staff. A practical benefit has been the facilitation of interlibrary loans between the Health Sciences and main USC campus. Many days have been saved by leaving loan requests on the board.

CONCLUSIONS

These activities can be put into perspective, to see what relevance they have for that new subject heading, LIBRARIAN-PATRON RELATIONS, and to see how the teaching of computer literacy is a natural and desirable continuation of the bibliographic skills that librarians have always taught to library users.[11] There is no doubt in the minds of Norris librarians that they have helped patrons to help themselves. The proof is there:

- successful seminar participants check out software;
- searchers have obtained NLM codes;
- the CD-ROM station is so popular that a reservation system was established to deal with the demand;
- statistics on usage of the microcomputer laboratory show steady growth and the computer assistant's hours have been increased 50 percent;

- software manufacturers have told librarians that patrons have purchased their programs upon the library's recommendation; producers continue to send updates and free copies of programs;
- patrons come back to tell librarians of programs they have discovered and to share experiences;
- librarians are invited to act as microcomputer consultants both on and off campus.

For the patron: the library is a place to meet, to learn, to hear about the latest in computer technology, and to discuss developments with members of other departments. Librarians can and will discuss hardware and software, assist in choosing appropriate programs, and arrange training and orientation sessions.

For the librarian: initial success in teaching online searching and reprint file management, organizing computer user groups, and automating internal office applications has led to the existence of the extensive facilities and programs described above. Computer expertise has widened librarians' vision of the information needs of users, enabled them to teach and consult, increased their awareness of the research being conducted on the campus, and facilitated relationships with faculty, staff, and researchers with whom they may not otherwise have come into contact.

For LIBRARIAN-PATRON RELATIONS: these have increased, broadened, and deepened. More patrons now have more contact on more levels with librarians who are able to help them in more ways. Mutual respect, understanding, and friendship have resulted from the exchange of computer skills.

Norris has not studied the possibility that seminar attendees, bulletin board callers, or computer user group members increase their use of books or journals. A library user is no longer defined only as someone who checks out a book or browses through journals. Microcomputers complement and supplement the access to information that the library provides. The skills needed to use the new technology (i.e., "computer literacy") are therefore taught by information specialists–librarians. Norris librarians are now participating more fully and actively in the overall educational and research missions of the university and are not only collectors and providers of the materials housed in the library, but have a much wider understanding of the world of information. Technological advances have produced a new kind of librarian, who relates to a new kind of patron.

One may ask whether patrons are aware that the library has contributed so much to their skills, and what this has done for the library's efficacy and its role in the academic community. A study on attitudes and views between librarians and patrons could be conducted, to see how they have changed as a result of the kind of interactions that this article has described. Meanwhile, at the Norris Medical Library, there is no doubt that teaching computer literacy has helped patrons to help themselves.

REFERENCES

1. Piele, L. I.; Pryor, J.; and Tuckett, H. W. "Teaching Microcomputer Literacy: New Roles for Academic Librarians." *College & Research Libraries* 47(July 1986):374-378.

2. Clark, K. *Civilisation.* New York: Harper and Row, 1969, p. 17.

3. Allegri, F. "Editorial Comment: What Is Information Literacy?" *Medical Reference Services Quarterly* 6(Spring 1987):95-97.

4. Dewey, M. "Preparation for the Library School." *Library Notes* 1(March 1987):272.

5. Friends, L. "Identifying and Informing the Potential End-User: *Online* Information Seminars." *Online* 10(January 1986):47-56.

6. Hubbard, A. "An Integrated Information Management Education Program . . . Defining a New Role for Librarians in Helping End-Users." *Online* 10(March 1986):15-23.

7. Arnold, S. E. "End-Users: Dreams or Dollars." *Online* 11(January 1987):71-81.

8. ACRL/BIS Task Force on Model Statement of Objectives. "Model Statement of Objectives for Academic Bibliographic Instruction: Draft Revision." *College & Research Libraries News* 48(May 1987):256-271.

9. Bennett, K. J.; Sackett, D. L.; Haynes, R. B.; Neufeld, V. R.; Tugwell, P.; and Roberts, R. "A Controlled Trial of Teaching Critical Appraisal of the Clinical Literature to Medical Students." *JAMA* 257(May 8, 1987):2451-2454.

10. Brown, J. F., and Wood, E. H. "Library-Sponsored Computer User Groups." *Bulletin of the Medical Library Association* 75(April 1987):167-169.

11. Kupferberg, N. "End-Users: How Are They Doing? A Librarian Interviews Six 'Do-It-Yourself' Searchers." *Online* 10(March 1986):24-28.

Chapter 21

The Librarian as Consultant and Educator for Personal File Management Software

Kathleen Strube
Carol M. Antoniewicz
Jacqueline Glick
Glynis Vandoorne Asu

It is a natural extension of the librarian's increasingly computer-oriented information managing skills to act as consultant to his or her institution concerning personal file management (PFM) software. PFM software automates and greatly improves a physician's or researcher's manual system of filing and managing a reprint collection. These personal collections of medical literature are often depended upon as a primary information source. Northrup's 1983 study concluded that, "because the personal library is the first line of resource (and possibly the only one in more rural areas), students need to be educated to create and maintain personal libraries and reprint files."[1] The microcomputer-based approach to personal file management is a relatively recent development and one that should definitely be attractive to those who publish in their fields and to those who attempt to create their own personalized subset of the medical literature. It is natural for the librarian rather than for others, such as an institution's computer department staff, to teach PFM skills because automated PFM represents the next step in information management after the forte of medical librarians–the MEDLINE search. Teaching computer-aided skills to store and ma-

This chapter was first published in *Medical Reference Services Quarterly*, Vol. 8(1), Spring 1989.

nipulate subsets of the medical literature is a logical follow-up for medical librarians who are already consulted to create the subsets.

Choosing a single system for reprint management can be confusing and time-consuming. The purpose of this chapter is to encourage librarians to learn more about PFM software and to take on the role of consultant, publicizer, and educator concerning this new technology for their institutions. Librarians can provide a welcome solution to the problem of the scientist's impossibly overgrown or unorganized personal reprint filing system, and publicize their skills as modern information technologists at the same time.

HISTORICAL OVERVIEW

Many articles in the literature emphasize the value of automating unwieldy manual reprint files.[2-10] Specialized database software for reprint management has been marketed commercially and successfully since the early 1980s. Before that time, there were a small number of health professionals, also computer enthusiasts, who wrote their own programs and ran them on large and expensive data-processing equipment.[11] Newer versions of the PFM programs from the early 1980s, now widely sold for use on personal microcomputers, are more flexible, have increased capabilities, and are easier to use. Advantages of PFM software over manual filing systems include downloading capabilities, increased access points for retrieval, and the abilities to insert in-text references in manuscripts and to compile bibliographies in the style of particular journals.

CAPABILITIES OF PFM SOFTWARE

PFM software programs can accept downloaded database searches, such as a MEDLINE search, eliminating the need to retype references. Some programs have telecommunications and menu-driven searching modules that allow users to perform their own searches prior to downloading into their personal files.

Searching an automated reprint file is more effective than searching a manual file because of increased access points. Balaban notes that, "reprints filed by subject (in a manual file) may not be quickly or accurately retrievable, because they could be filed under several equally appropriate subject headings."[12] There is virtually no limit to the number of subject headings that can be used for retrieval in a good PFM software program. Access is usually available by author, truncated author, truncated subject heading, truncated title word, journal name, or by any other string of characters entered in the record. For the publishing scientist or the support staff involved, good PFM software also banishes the need to retype bibliographies and in-text references when submitting a paper to a different journal (which of course requires a different format!). A few keystrokes can usually change the output from one style to another.

THE MCW EXPERIENCE

The Medical College of Wisconsin (MCW) Libraries reference staff began offering information on PFM software in 1986. Classes were given in which a member of the faculty who had several years experience using REF-11 shared his experience and gave advice on features to look for when purchasing PFM software. The reference staff secured demonstration copies of BOOKENDS, JOURNAL LOG, DATA FACTS, PC-FILE, REFERENCE MANAGER, SCI-MATE, PRO-CITE, and REF-11 for attendees to try. Promotional literature and a bibliography of articles on managing reprint collections were provided.

In 1987 reference staff decided to invest the time necessary to become experts on four PFM software products rather than depending on the schedules and availability of faculty members to speak at classes given in the Library. This desire to expand the user education program of MCW Libraries in the direction of more classes on information management is consistent with the goals of the Library. MCW Libraries wished to demonstrate that its own staff had computer expertise useful for solving the problems of personal file management. Reference staff wanted to offer regular classes and be available for walk-in consultations. Four PFM software products (SCI-MATE, PRO-CITE, REFERENCE MANAGER, and ASK-SAM) were chosen because they were mentioned most favorably in the literature, were most often asked for by interested faculty, and because library staff members had been impressed with the programs from demonstration copies used the year before (see Appendix for addresses of these four programs). The goal was to learn the programs well enough to demonstrate their use, and consequently to be able to compare the products and truly act as advisors and consultants to Medical College of Wisconsin faculty, staff, and students.

To encourage interest in PFM software in advance, articles were published in the library newsletter and in other institutional publications. Promotional brochures were made available near the circulation desk. This prompted many interested calls and questions. One specific result was that the Biochemistry Department asked that a reference librarian attend one of their department meetings to recommend a PFM system.

After interest had been heightened through publicity and expertise had been acquired during several months of working with the programs, planning was undertaken to create a formal educational program. The goals of teaching a class on PFM software were: (1) to promote greater awareness of the benefits of automating manual filing systems; (2) to compare the capabilities and limitations of four of the leading PFM software programs; and (3) to demonstrate the use of the four systems, including entering records by keyboard and by downloading, searching the PFM database, creating bibliographies in the formats required by several journals, and working with manuscripts to insert in-text references.

The class was scheduled to be two hours in length and was held in the Microdata Center of the Library. The class began with an introduction to PFM software and a comparison of the advantages of automated versus manual systems. A discussion followed comparing capabilities of each of the four software programs using a visual aid in the form of a chart (see Table 21.1) drawn up by the reference librarians that compared the four programs. Results listed in the chart rate SCI-MATE as the most difficult program to learn as well as having the most complicated process for downloading the results of database searches. REFERENCE MANAGER is rated the easiest to master in those respects. ASKSAM is unlike the other three programs in that it was created for more purposes than just reprint management. With ASKSAM, input can be very simple and unstructured; however, with this type of input, output in different journal styles is not available. With an optional module, REF-ERENCE MANAGER offers the output styles required by 100 different journals. PRO-CITE offers 20 different workforms for 20 different document types, the largest number of preset workforms of these four programs. Discounts are available for quantity purchases or through institutional programs, making the prices of the four pieces of software very comparable.

Twenty- to 30-minute demonstrations of the four systems followed discussion of the comparative chart. Software demonstrations were projected on a screen with an Electrohome projector. Handouts included the comparative chart, a list of faculty members already using a PFM program and willing to answer questions, promotional literature, and recent articles about the various programs.

The class, limited to ten people because of room size, attracted primarily support staff of faculty members, specifically secretaries or research assistants. Only one attendee was a faculty member. This is not meant to suggest that support staff are the only audience for this type of class. However, at the Medical College of Wisconsin, faculty members requested alternatives to attending a formal class. They preferred to learn about PFM software or about specific programs by calling the Library, by coming into the Library individually, or by having a librarian attend a departmental meeting.

DISCUSSION

Parts of the class that worked well for attendees were the initial presentation of the value and capabilities of PFM software, and the discussion of the feature-by-feature comparisons in the chart. A definite problem with the class was that the half-hour demonstrations of each piece of software were too long for an educational experience that intended to introduce and compare, but not long enough for the purpose of mastering use of a particular program. Several attendees left after watching the demonstration of the PFM program in which they were most interested and others appeared restless or bored during portions of the demonstrations.

The Electrohome projector that was used to demonstrate the four

TABLE 21.1. A Comparison of Four File Management Software Programs

	SCI-MATE 2.0/2.1	ASKSAM 4.0	PRO-CITE 1.3	REFERENCE MANAGER 4.0
PRICE	$384 w/MCW discount	$240 w/MCW discount	$395 quantity discounts available	$440 quantity discounts available: $40-$50 add.mods.
HARDWARE	IBM	IBM	IBM MAC	IBM KAYPRO DEC MAC soon
READABLE EXTERNAL FILES	Must search with Sci-Mate SEARCHER Works w/Word-Star or Word-Perfect Reads Dialog, BRS, NLM, ASCII ‡D‡	Reads any ASCII file No telecom. software included ‡M‡	Reads Dialog, BRS, NLM, MUMS, SCORPIO, OCLC, RLIN, NOTIS w/Biblio-Links ‡E‡ works in conjunction w/WP thru ASCII	Reads MEDLINE files from NLM, BRS, DIALOG, PAPER-CHASE, Grateful Med/BIOSIS Works w/WordStar WordPerf, XYWrite Microsoft Word Edix/Wordix. ASCII ‡E‡
‡ REFERENCES HANDLED (F = FLOPPY H = HARD DISK)	F = 500-1000 H = 64 User Files 32767 records/file	Capacity limited only by size of floppy or hard disk used	F = 700 H = 30,000	F=750/360Kb H=25,000/10MB

‡E‡ = Easy to do or learn
‡M‡ = Moderately easy (Takes several steps or some persistence to accomplish)
‡D‡ = Difficult to do or learn (Takes a great deal of effort & time)

TYPES OF REF'S HANDLED	Books Journals Can create others	5 Types Books, Journals, Chapters, etc. Can create others	20 Types	6 Types Books, Journals, Chapters, Slides w/ add. nod.
BOOLEAN LOGIC?	yes	yes also arithmetic: if-then-else	yes	yes
PRINT REF'S W/O WP?	yes	yes	yes	yes
REORDERS AUTHORS: (SURNAME + INITIALS?)	yes	yes	yes new in ver. 1.3	yes
DICTIONARY FILE OF KEYWORDS CREATED?	no	not automatic, is possible	not automatic, is possible	yes author, keyword
U = UNDERLINE S = SUB, SUPERSCRIPT B = BOLD, I = ITALICS	U,B,I	U,B	U,B	U,I,B,S,SUP
HOW EASY TO LEARN?	‡D‡	‡M‡	‡M‡	‡E‡

TABLE 21.1 (continued)

	SCI-MATE 2.0/2.1	ASKSAM 4.0	PRO-CITE 1.3	REFERENCE MANAGER 4.0
‡ OUTPUT STYLES, J FORMATS?	15	None	8	3 incl., 10 add. disk
CAN OTHER OUTPUT STYLES BE CREATED?	yes	with ‡M‡ difficulty	yes	yes
COORDINATE W/REF #'S IN MANUSCRIPT?	yes	no	yes	yes
PHONE SUPPORT?	Good toll-free	Good not toll-free	Good not toll-free	Good toll-free
DOCUMENTATION?	‡D‡ minimal help screens 3 vol. doc.	‡ not reviewed indexed manual w/9 lessons help screens	‡M‡ help screens	‡E‡ help screens abound

PFM programs on a large screen was not consistently clear and totally obscured any line that was highlighted. This greatly reduced the effectiveness of the demonstrations and may have led to some of the symptoms of short attention span.

FUTURE DIRECTIONS

To improve future group classes, the reference staff plans to purchase a new projector and offer a shorter introduction-and-comparison seminar, describing the pros and cons of several PFM software programs. Attendees, or anyone with an interest, will be able to make individual appointments for demonstrations. Another option will be that groups will be able to request a class on any one particular program. Librarians will continue to act as consultants by attending department meetings or by demonstrating particular programs in the reference department of the Library.

Evaluation of progress to date in attempting to educate library staff and the Medical College of Wisconsin in general to the benefits of PFM software has led to the following conclusions. Learning to use PFM software has definitely been worthwhile for the Library in terms of public relations and image enhancement. Reference librarians *are* able to act as consultants to their institution's concerning this time-saving new technology. Aggressively providing direction and guidance for the all-too-common faculty problem of how to manage overgrown reprint files enhances the library's image as an organization of professionals with computer and information management skills. Benefits to the institution whose library offers this type of training include greater numbers of faculty and staff who can more efficiently find, manipulate, and publish information.

APPENDIX

SCI-MATE 2.0/2.1
ISI Software Tech. Sup.
3501 Market St.
Philadelphia, PA 19104
800-523-4092

ASKSAM 4.0
Seaside Software
119 S. Washington St.
P.O. Box 1428
Perry, FL 32347
800-327-5726

PRO-CITE 1.3
Personal Bibliographic
Software Inc.
412 Longshore Dr.
Ann Arbor, MI 48105
313-996-1580

REFERENCE MANAGER 4.0
Research Information Inc. (RIS)
Suite 206
Encinitas, CA 92042
800-722-1227

REFERENCES

1. Northrup, D.E. "Characteristics of Clinical Information-Searching: Investigation Using Critical Incident Technique." *Journal of Medical Education* 58(1983):873-881.

2. Golden, W.E., and Friedlander, I.R. "Students Evaluate MEDFILE, a Preprinted Medical Literature Filing System." *Medical Education* 21(1987):314-319.

3. Gurney, Jud W., and Wigton, Robert S. "Computerized Reference Management–Filing the Literature."*AJR* 149(August 1987):411-413.

4. Haynes, R. Brian; McKibbon, Ann K.; Fitzgerald, Dorothy; Guyatt, Gordon, H.; Walker, Cynthia J.; and Sackett, David L. "How to Keep Up with the Medical Literature: VI. How to Store and Retrieve Articles Worth Keeping." *Annals of Internal Medicine* 105(1986):978-984.

5. Hedden, Judy. "Sci-Mate and Searcher's Tool Kit: A Comparative Review." *Database End-User* (December 1986):18-26.

6. Hoyle, Norman. "Biblio-Link and Pro-Cite: The Searcher's Workstation." *Database* 10(February 1987):73-78.

7. Hubbard, Abigail. "Reprint File Management Software." *Online* 9(November 1985):67-73.

8. Pruett, Nancy Jones. "Using AskSam to Manage Files of Bibliographic References." *Online* 11(July 1987):46-52.

9. Schmid, K., and Bohmer, G. "Reference Master: A Microcomputer-Based Storage and Retrieval System for Bibliographic References." *International Journal of Bio-Medical Computing* 20(1987):107-121.

10. Wachtel, Ruth E. "Personal Bibliographic Databases." *Science* 235(February 27, 1987):1093-1096.

11. Bjoraker, David G. "Experience with Microcomputer Management of a Personal Medical Literature Collection." *Journal of Medical Systems* 8(1984): 103-110.

12. Balaban, Donald J.; Wright, Gail K.; Innes, Frank T.; and Goldfarb, Neil I. "Choosing a Micro Database for Easy Retrieval of Reprints." *MD Computing* 4(1987):23-29.

Chapter 22

Building a Clinical Consulting Program

Mitchell Aaron Cahan

In January 1989, the William H. Welch Medical Library of the Johns Hopkins University School of Medicine established a personal information management program. As part of its commitment to integrated academic information management in a decentralized environment, the library focuses its educational efforts on teaching the conceptual and technological skills necessary to exploit modern bibliographic information systems in biomedicine. This chapter presents a preliminary overview of the process of launching a novel consulting program in a clinical environment.

BACKGROUND

Welch serves a campus that ranks among the top three universities nationally in federal funding for biomedical research. The Johns Hopkins Medical Institutions (JHMI) consists of several academic divisions including the School of Medicine, School of Hygiene and Public Health, School of Nursing, and the Johns Hopkins Hospital. Two Ethernet high speed networks link a variety of computing facilities throughout the campus. The networks support clinical, research, and literature retrieval systems. The library's computerized information retrieval system, WELMED, allows researchers to search the biomedical literature and request photocopies of documents from the laboratory, office, or ward.

This chapter was first published in *Medical Reference Services Quarterly*, Vol. 9(1), Spring 1990.

In a recent planning effort, Welch staff identified consulting as an objective in the library's strategic plan. The plan calls for the development of a program to promote information management throughout the campus. Consulting focuses on the adoption of information technology for successful information management at both a personal and a departmental level. True integration of information management within the clinical setting would result from a proactive program designed to teach skills within the hospital and research environment. Since 1988 Welch librarians have contacted JHMI department chairmen offering an overview of Welch services and descriptions of relevant areas of the collection. The librarians have also solicited advice on collection development. Although the idea of a consulting program evolved out of the library's educational mission, the concept of personal information management provides an individualized approach that a series of scheduled information management education (IME) classes does not offer. The consulting program supports clients in many of the same areas taught in IME sessions but differs from them by structuring the presentation around a specialized clinical area. IME sessions usually occur in the library setting while personalized information management sessions usually take place in the hospital. The consulting approach emphasizes a tailored program designed to meet the information needs of an individual or an entire subspecialty. Thus, IME and tailored consulting coexist, providing separate but equally important areas of library service.

Although knowledge of the information needs of clinical workers remains incomplete, Welch staff have identified a series of information management skills of direct relevance for the health care worker. For the first phase of the program, the consulting service provides support for:

Technologies: Networking, Telecommunications Software, Microcomputing, HyperCard® Programming
Information Retrieval: Hopkins Current Contents,® Search Strategy Construction, WELMED, BRS Colleague, Physician Data Query, Grateful MED®
Information Processing: Reprint Management, Database Construction, Thesaurus Construction

With the establishment of the program, the consulting coordinator identified expertise among the Welch staff and assigned areas of responsibility to each librarian. The scope of the consulting program evolved from questions received at the information desk, requests for extensive assistance from library clientele, and topics covered in IME programs.

ADMINISTRATION

The coordinator drafted a mission statement, identified the scope of the program, and centralized the consulting process to provide for a manageable work load for all librarians. The coordinator also developed consulting procedures, established statistical records, and created an educational program for staff. Next, the coordinator attempted to identify potential consulting opportunities in a systematic fashion. For example, the Dean for Research of the School of Medicine now describes the consulting program in his initial correspondence to all new faculty members, a copy of which he sends to the consulting coordinator. Other contacts have resulted from following up leads seen in newsletters of the various divisions of the JHMI. A major effort will involve the creation of an organizational chart so clinical personnel can be contacted regularly.

The coordinator identified a protocol for handling consulting requests. Staff librarians are responsible for consulting session logistics. These procedures include:

- Identify the information needs of the department or individual;
- Survey the number and type of equipment and network facilities;
- Ensure adequacy of facilities for presentation;
- Schedule and transport equipment to the site;
- Prepare packets (some clerical support provided);
- Submit a written report for review by Welch librarians;
- Conduct follow-up as needed.

A statistics sheet is used to document each session. The form tracks the client's name, affiliation, interests, and plans for follow-up. For group sessions, clients record their name and telephone number, allowing for follow-up when necessary. A library assistant tabulates the statistics on a monthly basis. The report circulates to all members of the library's management team to help them monitor the needs of library clientele and allocate resources.

Due to the demand for consulting services, no single individual can respond to every request for personal information management services. As a result, the coordinator depends on the skills of an entire staff. Although most requests for consulting services originate with the coordinator, the program relies on the skills of seven professionals. The coordinator devised a form to keep staff current on the latest developments in information technology. Although originally intended for those involved in the consulting program, the staff education series has evolved into a continuing education program for all interested staff in the library. Approximately 20 librarians and reference assistants participate in the staff education program at one or more levels. Every staff member working with library clientele, in the consulting program or in the context of reference services, needs a minimal level of knowledge of all core consulting areas. In addition, librarians require competence at a basic level of knowledge in all areas that fall under the scope of the program. At a third level, each librarian has chosen an area of expertise which requires mastering all aspects of a subject, keeping abreast of changes in the area, and authoring publications and presenting papers. Grateful MED® serves as an example of the various layers of knowledge inculcated in the staff education program. At the awareness level, library assistants know that Grateful MED® serves as one of the most inexpensive, user-friendly programs for searching MEDLINE. Librarians, working at a basic level of understanding, appreciate the scope of the package and know how to teach it. The expert has a mastery of all aspects, including the Grateful MED® search engine, and conducts research on Grateful MED® as a tool for searching the literature. An expert's final responsibility involves conducting educational sessions for staff on a weekly basis in support of staff consulting activities. A list of topics offered during 1989 included:

- Janus: The Online Catalog of the Johns Hopkins University Milton S. Eisenhower Library
- Grateful MED®
- BRS Colleague

- Communications Software for the Macintosh
- Communications Software for the IBM
- Molecular Biology Databases
- Apple on the Leading Edge
- HyperCard®
- Reprint Management Packages
- Virus Detection and Eradication
- Smartcom and Reference Manager
- Nursing Information Resources
- Facsimile Transmission
- Introduction to Unix
- Bibliographic Verification using SERLINE and CATLINE: A Practical Approach
- Micromesh

Librarians share responsibility for conducting these sessions. Sometimes guest lecturers from outside of the institution participate. Classes are offered using a lecture or hands-on approach. Some classes are repeated due to importance for library clientele.

CONSULTING IN THE CLINICAL ENVIRONMENT

Personal information management in the clinical setting combines both an educational and a service orientation. Although superficially similar to clinical medical librarianship of the last 15 years, the library consultant does more than transfer the reference desk beyond the walls of the library. Consulting demands learning on the part of both the information specialist and the client. In order to master the information needs of a clinical department, the library consultant must gain some degree of familiarity with the latest research and clinical concerns of the department in question. The client, on the other hand, agrees to learn about information technologies as a tool for improving patient care in the hospital setting. No longer does the clinical librarian act as a "pair-of-hands" for the clinical worker; instead, skills gained through the consulting session allow clients to begin to manage their own information needs. For example, based on the skills gained from a previous consulting session, a clinician may identify several relevant review articles on mitral stenosis by searching Grateful MED® and download the citations into Reference Manager® without requiring the assistance of a librarian.

The success of consulting in a clinical area of the campus largely revolves around identification of a supportive sponsor. A sponsor usually has an administrative position in the department and can legitimize the consulting activity. Consulting activities may arise from solicitation by the consulting coordinator or upon request by a member of the JHMI faculty, staff, or student body. An initial conversation with the sponsor usually provides the consultant with an idea of the client's information needs. After agreeing on a time and place (usually the clinical setting), the consultant prepares materials of direct interest to the client. An initial session may last up to two hours. The first consulting opportunity usually focuses on the library's information systems, including WELMED and Hopkins Current Contents.® Depending on the interests of the department, additional sessions may examine fee-based information services such as Grateful MED® or BRS Colleague. Many clinical workers request a demonstration of a reprint management package. In its first six months, the program has assisted over 20 clinical departments.

CAVEATS AND CONCLUSIONS

A librarian planning to establish a personal information management program should not expect immediate changes in the information-seeking patterns of its clientele. For example, the limited Welch experience demonstrates that many clients do not have adequate access to computer hardware in the clinical setting. As a result, many of those individuals seen in the clinical environment cannot take advantage of electronic information services. One solution to the problem of hardware access might involve the creation of a loaner program for temporary support of a department's hardware needs prior to purchase of requisite equipment.

Another observation during the early months of the program is that true mastery of an information technology requires more than a single consulting session. Practice is an essential ingredient in conceptual learning; practice necessitates a substantial commitment of time, often difficult for the busy practitioner. In addition, consulting requires substantial staff resources. For instance, during the first six months of the program, without much promotion of the program, staff spent approximately 475 hours consulting with 533 clients. A one-hour consulting session may require from five minutes to ten hours of preparation depending on the complexity of the topic. Present levels of consulting activities have pushed an already taxed staff to its limits. Moreover, the fluid nature of technology requires that the consulting program evolve as the nature of information management changes. The scope of the program must adapt to the changing needs of library clientele.

Despite the amount of work involved in operating a consulting program, the concept of personalized information management may play a critical role in supporting integrated information management in the academic, biomedical setting. The novelty of the program precludes definitive answers regarding the efficacy of personal information management consulting. Currently a plan is being prepared that will address the future course of the program including assessment of its impact on JHMI. In the meantime, information specialists will increasingly work throughout the campus promoting information technologies. With the assistance of the consulting librarian, much meaningful learning can take place in the familiar environs of the clinic, lab, or office.

Chapter 23

Introducing Computer Literacy Skills for Physicians

Barbara Collins
Anne Linton
Jonathan Merril
Karyn Pomerantz
Sally Winthrop

Physicians require information to support patient care decisions and to conduct research. The American Association of Medical Colleges (AAMC) has recognized the importance of training physicians in medical informatics,[1] and many institutions are preparing their students and residents to use literature retrieval and medical decision support software.[2-4] Blonde and Guthrie have presented workshops on medical informatics for program directors and chairs of internal medicine departments at the American College of Physicians' "Teaching Internal Medicine" biannual meeting.[5] Ryan, Hayward, and Richardson are developing a curriculum to teach computerized information management skills to internal medicine residents at Johns Hopkins Hospital and Francis Scott Key Hospital in Baltimore.[6]

Some physicians have never been exposed to literature retrieval systems, file management programs, or presentation software during their medical training. Many academic health sciences libraries are taking the lead to change this situation. They offer classes in word processing, spreadsheet programs, and information retrieval skills. The Alfred Taubman Medical Library at the University of

This chapter was first published in *Medical Reference Services Quarterly*, Vol. 11(4), Winter 1992.

Michigan trained staff physicians to manage their reprint files,[7] and physicians have been a target population for end-user searching workshops at many health sciences libraries.[8-10]

The Himmelfarb Health Sciences Library at the George Washington University Medical Center sponsors a wide variety of computer and information management classes. However, few community physicians with hospital privileges at the Medical Center enroll. In order to reach this underserved group, often referred to as attendings, the Library and the Department of Computer Medicine of the George Washington University Medical Center presented a workshop, "Introducing Your Office Computer!" This workshop focused on the educational needs of the attending physician.

GOALS

"Introducing Your Office Computer!" was designed to achieve three goals. First, it introduced physicians to the various hardware and software options available to support their information needs. The workshop was introductory and broad-based. Teaching specific skills was not an objective of the program. Instructors hoped that physicians, new to the world of personal computers, would leave the workshop eager to explore some of the options presented.

A second objective involved introducing attendees to Library services, particularly educational services. Himmelfarb Library offers its educational programs and computer facilities to all physicians with privileges at the University hospital. Therefore, microcomputer classes, consultation services, and instructional software available in the Audiovisual Study Center were highlighted throughout the workshop as a means of learning in detail about the topics covered.

Finally, on an organizational level, the Library staff wanted to build a closer relationship with the Department of Computer Medicine. Members of the Department are skilled in computer-assisted instruction and the role of computers in medical practice. Their participation added credibility and depth to the workshop.

SCOPE

The workshop highlighted computer applications for clinical research, education, and patient care. Topics reviewed included modems, graphic cards, electronic mail, literature searching, computer-aided diagnosis, and presentation software. To provide a framework that attendees could use to assess each software package, the planning committee of librarians and a physician wrote a case history about a patient with colon cancer. This simulation provided the basis for a search question, a slide, etc.

Office software used for billing, medical history-taking, or patient scheduling was outside of the scope of this program. Copies of articles and a bibliography on those topics were provided.

MARKETING

Two major approaches were used to publicize this workshop. An announcement was included in the Library's fall calendar of courses that is distributed to physicians on the faculty. Several physicians enrolled soon after receiving their calendars.

To reach more physicians in a personalized way, letters were mailed six weeks prior to the workshop to 150 attending physicians, physicians in private practice who have hospital privileges but are not located on the university campus. The letter stressed the introductory nature of the program and reassured applicants that no computer skills were necessary. These letters generated an immediate response. Ten physicians enrolled within one week of receiving the letters. An upper limit of 25 attendees was established to allow personal attention. The planning committee did not expect a registration above this limit.

Marketing continued with posters placed in the physicians' lounge in the University hospital and with an announcement in a newsletter produced by the Medical Center's public relations department. A final tally of 12 people registered. Consultations with a librarian were offered to people who could not attend, and two were scheduled. A $25.00 fee was charged for the workshop.

ATTENDEES

Of the 12 physicians who registered for the workshop, all but one attended. Four were senior physicians in the community with many years of experience. Seven were younger physicians with an average of 15 to 20 years of practice experience. They represented various medical specialties, including urology, thoracic surgery, gastroenterology, general internal medicine, and neurology. All admitted to only a superficial familiarity with computers and information technology.

FORMAT: INFORMATION FAIR

The workshop was scheduled from 1:30 PM to 4:00 PM on a Wednesday afternoon. It was organized as a "fair" with five computer stations set up around the room to introduce specific applications and provide hands-on experience with software programs. Each station was staffed by a librarian or physician from the Department of Computer Medicine.

Originally, the organizers arranged to have the participants listen to five 20-minute lecture/demonstrations of various computer applications. However, they decided that it would be difficult to hold the attention of the participants using a purely didactic format. It was decided to allow attendees to personalize their instruction and to learn by doing.

A casual and relaxed atmosphere was maintained. Coffee and cookies were available. Many participants knew each other, contributing to the friendly atmosphere.

A librarian opened the workshop by stating the goals and expectation that this would be an introductory session which required no prior knowledge. Packets containing a bibliography of books and articles on computer applications in medicine and selected articles on choosing computer hardware and software were distributed. Evaluation forms and an invitation for a second session in the spring were also included. Attendees were asked to pass this invitation along to colleagues, thus providing another avenue of publicity for the spring workshop.

A representative from the Department of Computer Medicine, addressed the group next and discussed the role of computer-assisted learning and testing programs in contemporary medical education. He played a videotape demonstrating specific programs. This generated interest and discussion about the role of computerized programs in medical practice and education. People were interested in the variety of compact disc products and in comparisons of computer-based testing with conventional methods.

After this presentation, the group divided into teams of two or three to circulate among the five computer stations arranged around the periphery of the room.

Each station displayed a separate application on a stand-alone personal computer. Because the University supports an IBM environment, the hardware and software used for instructional purposes are IBM-based. The computers were those available in the Library's Microcomputer Lab and classroom. They ranged from old XTs with black and white monitors that were used to demonstrate searching and electronic mail to newer 386 machines with color monitors that were used to show presentation software, Windows, and the diagnostic support program. The newer ones were equipped with a keyboard and a mouse.

The applications were:

- Microsoft DOS and Microsoft Windows for organizing a computer,
- Software Publishing Company's Harvard Graphics for presenting information on slides,
- The Library's electronic mail system, BITNET, and the Internet for communicating with colleagues,
- MEDLINE on BRS/Colleague and miniMEDLINE™ for literature searching,
- DxPLAIN for diagnostic decision-making support.

Reference librarians or a Computer Medicine physician staffed each station and demonstrated the system's capabilities. They also distributed additional handouts on specific subjects such as DOS commands, telecommunications software, and Grateful MED and BRS/Colleague. Questions were entertained at each station. The physicians inquired about modem selection, differences between DOS and Windows, and the mechanics of searching. They were encouraged to try their hands on the computer and to move on to other stations as needed. Several toured the Audiovisual Study Center and experimented with additional instructional software there following the workshop.

No physician volunteered to use the computer during the demonstrations. They preferred watching and guiding the instructors' inputs into the computers. This is an issue that will be addressed before future workshops are offered.

FEEDBACK

The responses were overwhelmingly positive. Even before the session was held, several physicians called to verify the content of the program and expressed gratitude for the Library's efforts.

At the program's conclusion, the attendees unanimously expressed their appreciation, calling the afternoon fun and stimulating. Two members of a Medical Society committee discussed how they could start using the Library's electronic mail system, Mail-Man, to communicate with committee members.

Although only one attendee returned the written evaluation form, several physicians called the Library to make arrangements to use Library databases. One of the physicians in this class attended a subsequent program on medical informatics. Another wanted more opportunity to try the programs demonstrated. He wrote:

> Instructors tend to use the machines and students tend to shy away and let them. The reverse should be encouraged.

Another physician requested Continuing Medical Education credits for the workshop. Recognizing this as a factor important to physicians, Category I CME credits were granted for the spring workshop.

EVALUATION

The instructors were also very pleased with the program. They felt that the workshop filled a need in the physician community and were gratified by the responses received.

Strengths of the program included the personalized presentations at the computer stations and the contributions of each staff member. Because each person was responsible for only a segment of the workshop, there was minimal preparation time needed to compile handouts and practice presentations. One of the librarian instructors coordinated the arrangements for marketing, signage, catering, name tags, and information packets. Approximately ten hours total time was needed to prepare the workshop. The joint efforts strengthened team spirit and the relationship between the Library and the Department of Computer Medicine.

Improvements are planned for the spring session. The opening segment on computer-based training and decision making will be extended to an hour to permit more questions and discussion. A CD-ROM station will be substituted for the DOS/Windows demonstration. To encourage more participation at each station, instructors will present a problem and guide the physicians in solving it. By the end of the workshop, instructors expect each participant to create a slide, send an E-mail message, enter a search online and on compact disc, and make a differential diagnosis.

Individual follow-up needs to be conducted after the session. Each participant can be called to elicit any new questions or requests for consultations.

SUMMARY

"Introducing Your Office Computer!" provided a valuable introduction to information management skills to attending physicians at The George Washington University Medical Center. The computer fair format provided variety and personal attention. Participants and instructors rated the experience highly. For the next workshop, there will be more time to discuss innovations in medical informatics and increased emphasis on hands-on experimentation. It has been a rewarding experience for the Library staff as well as for the physicians.

REFERENCES

1. Steering Committee on the Evaluation of Medical Information Science in Medical Education. "Evaluation of Medical Information Science in Medical Education: An Agenda for Action." *Journal of Medical Education* 61 (June 1986):193-500.

2. Wood E.H.; Morrison I.L.; and Oppenheimer P.R. "Drug Information Skills for Pharmacy Students: Curriculum Integration." *Bulletin of the Medical Library Association* 78 (January 1990):8-14.

3. Bradigan, P.S., and Mularski, C.A. "End-User Searching in a Medical School Curriculum: An Evaluated Modular Approach." *Bulletin of the Medical Library Association* 77 (October 1989):348-356.

4. Broering, N.C. "The MAClinical Workstation Project at Georgetown University." *Bulletin of the Medical Library Association* 79 (July 1991):276-281.

5. Blonde, L., and Guthrie, R.D., Jr. "Using Computers in Internal Medicine Education." Workshop presented at "Teaching Internal Medicine," conference sponsored by the American College of Physicians in Chicago on October 23, 1991.

6. Ryan, S.D.; Hayward, R.; and Richardson, J. "A Curriculum in Information Management for Internal Medicine Residents." October 1991. (Grant application from Ryan, S.D., Hayward, R., and Richardson, J. to Chesapeake Physicians Professional Assoc.)

7. Dow, S.C. "Teaching Reprint File Management: A Hands-On Approach." *Medical Reference Services Quarterly* 9 (Fall 1990):31-41.

8. Ginn, D.S.; Pinkowski, P.E.; and Tylman, W.T. "Evolution of an EndUser Training Program. *Bulletin of the Medical Library Association* 75 (April 1987): 117-121.

9. Wender, R.W. "Teaching MEDLINE to Non-Urban End Users." *Medical Reference Services Quarterly* 8 (Summer 1989):25-40.

10. Wannarka, M.B. "A Training Program for the End User in the Academic Health Sciences Center." *Medical Reference Services Quarterly* 5 (Summer 1986):95-101.

Chapter 24

Information Management Education for Students in the Health Care Professions: A Coordinated, Integrated Plan

Judy F. Burnham

INTRODUCTION

Information literacy may be defined as the ability to effectively access and evaluate information for problem solving and decision making. Information literate persons know how knowledge and information are organized, how to find various types of information, how to organize information, and how to use information in problem solving.[1]

Through information management (IM), an individual can achieve information literacy. In addition to furnishing the desired information, the goal of IM education is to teach methods of information collection that will assist students throughout their careers.[2] Information management should enable students to retrieve appropriate, dependable, complete information by efficiently using information resource tools, and thus develop the skills needed for lifelong learning.[3]

The information explosion in the field of health care has made it necessary for students in these disciplines to become active learners, not just recipients of information. Limited time does not allow

This chapter was first published in *Medical Reference Services Quarterly*, Vol. 13(2), Summer 1994.

instruction in all areas. Also, because these disciplines have a responsibility for lifelong learning, it is necessary for the students to
depend on the literature to gain the information needed for a given
situation.[4,5]

Information management can be offered as a separate class, or it
can be integrated into the present curriculum. Allegri states that
course-integrated instruction must meet three of the following four
criteria:

> (1) faculty outside the library are involved in the design,
> execution and evaluation of the program, (2) the instruction is
> curriculum-based, in other words, directly related to the stu-
> dents' course work and/or assignments, (3) students are re-
> quired to participate, and (4) the students' work is graded or
> credit is received for participation.[6]

IM education is most meaningful at the time of need when benefits
can best be seen, and the most effective IM programs are those that
are integrated into the coursework and have a required assignment.[7]
Explanation of how to use a resource tool right before a student is
required to write a paper will be more meaningful than presenting
the information during orientation the week before classes begin.

Curriculum integration of IM allows information-seeking to be
taught as a thinking process, with less emphasis on the end result.
Integration of IM enhances cognition and problem solving. The
result is that the student is able to incorporate the instruction into
future research, rather than use it only in that specific instance.

Elective classes reach only those students who can fit them into
their schedule, and are motivated to do so. But integrating IM into
the core curriculum classes assures that it will reach all of the
students.[4-8]

Suggested categories of courses which are suitable for integrating IM are those that: (1) concern research, (2) have a writing
component, (3) involve independent or directed study, (4) involve
problem-solving assignments, (5) involve preparation of a bibliography, or (6) involve patient management questions. Other categories can be identified by working with the curriculum committee in
each college.[4]

Integrating information management into a curriculum takes

planning and coordination to avoid gaps and overlap. The overall plan should be developed in conjunction with the administration of the colleges served. Key faculty from these colleges, as well as students, should work with the designated librarian to identify target classes and to identify the needs of the students. IM education provided by the library should not be restricted to the courses targeted by the coordinated program. Rather, it should be presented in additional courses when requested, and those courses considered for inclusion in the IM program.

Information management education should be a building process. Information given at the entry level is very basic, with more advanced information offered at the next levels. Each level builds on the previous ones.[9] General information on library services and policies needs to be included in the orientation process for all new students, focusing on arrangement, collection parameters, policies and procedures, services available, and an introduction to the staff. Orientation emphasizes making the user comfortable in the library.[10-13]

Each IM unit should include a statement of the user's instructional needs, written instructional objectives, and a statement concerning financial and staff support, with users (students, faculty, etc.) participating in the development and evaluation of each unit.[10] A questionnaire, analyzing the organization and instructional methods and materials, can be distributed to the students following each session.[15]

Faculty cooperation is necessary for the success of any information management program. There must be continuing and open communication between the librarians and the faculty so that changes in the students' information needs can be met.[9] Once established, the library component needs to be listed in the syllabus of the targeted course. Teaching methods for each unit could include lecture, demonstration, and/or seminar format. Use of instructional aids (overhead transparencies, slides, video, etc.) is encouraged, with handouts being used as appropriate. If possible, the source(s) under discussion should be brought to class so the students can review the materials.[16] An effective instructional method is to choose a topic relevant to the course and describe the steps necessary to research it with the resource tools covered.[17] A bibliography may also be appropriate.[14] A required and graded assignment using the information skills taught will help stress the importance of learning those skills. The assignment should be individualized and relevant, while not too time-consuming.

A pretest and a posttest should be prepared for each IM unit, to evaluate its effectiveness. If time permits, the librarian ought to visit the class a second time to give suggestions on improving the information search strategies conducted by the class.[18]

PROGRAM DEVELOPMENT

Before 1989, there was not an organized information management education program at the University of South Alabama. Library instruction was included in the classes of faculty members who were strong library users themselves, but was not included in others. The result was that some students received instruction during several different classes, while others received no information management instruction at all. As a result of this, a coordinated information management program was planned for the three colleges that the Biomedical Library serves.

After a search of the literature, a plan specifying that different skills be taught at different academic levels was created by an information services librarian. Each year would be a building block for the following year, avoiding gaps and overlap. The information management plan, with written objectives and a memo outlining implementation of the plan, was submitted to the Deans of the three colleges, with a request for feedback.

The librarian who designed the IM plan met with the Dean and department chairs of the College of Nursing. After discussion, minor revisions were made to better meet the requirements of the curriculum and the needs of the students, and a class at each academic level was targeted. With the Dean's support, contact was made with the instructors, and specific plans and objectives were designed for each class. Some classes include orientation/instruction in the library, some include lecture in the classroom, and some include both. Assignments are required for most classes.

The librarian also met with the Dean of the College of Allied Health Professions to discuss the proposal. Because of the curriculum design for the students in this college, IM education is currently a one-time opportunity, rather than being taught at each academic level. Three disciplines in the College–Physical Therapy, Respiratory Care and Cardiopulmonary Sciences, and Medical Technology–participate in a required research class that involves students from all three areas. When the plan was developed, the librarian, working with the coursemaster for the class, submitted a list of IM objectives to the faculty charged with designing the course, and revisions were made to the objectives based on the suggestions of those attending. The IM session includes both lecture in the classroom and demonstration in the library. The assignment for the class, a worksheet which accounts for 10 percent of the grade, requires that the students use tools covered in the library instruction to locate references on a topic related to the course.

Before the information management plan was adopted in the College of Medicine, there was little formal library instruction for the medical students. As curriculum changes in the College of Medicine must be approved by the Curriculum Committee, the librarian volunteered to serve and was appointed to the committee; this assisted in the presentation of the IM plan. Discussion of the plan at a committee meeting resulted in some positive changes to the plan and its adoption for the first three years of medical school. Because of the scheduling problems, the fourth-year medical students were not included.

Faculty cooperation has not been forthcoming in all targeted classes for the three disciplines. In those cases, other classes have been substituted, or the librarian has tried to work with the college or department. In all aspects of the creation of this plan, the librarian has found that it is best to work within the system, although this is sometimes time-consuming. Of course, information management is not limited to the targeted classes; sessions that focus on the course subject areas are added when requested by professors. If skills are needed before they are taught in a group setting, the librarian instructs one-on-one. Classes consist of either classroom lecture or demonstration in the library, depending on the needs of the class and the preference of the instructor. Examples used are relevant to that class. Following each IM session, evaluations are completed by the students, with plans underway to analyze the evaluations using a computerized statistical program. Revisions are made in the IM plan each quarter, reflecting changes in curriculum, new technologies available, and successes and/or failures of the previous quarter.

PROGRAM DESCRIPTIONS

College of Nursing

IM for the nursing students is treated as a building process. Below is a list of the general objectives of information management for the undergraduate students in that discipline.[11,17,19-21]

An awareness of:

- the physical arrangement of the library and library services provided
- strategies for current awareness
- statistical sources
- Grateful MED
- reprint management programs
- citation indexing
- sources available using the Internet

The ability to:

- determine the location of materials using an online catalog
- use major nursing and medical reference sources and text-books
- use CINAHL (printed and CD-ROM)
- use *Index Medicus* and MEDLINE
- use indexing and abstracting services and online systems in the health sciences
- use indexing and abstracting services and online systems in other disciplines
- formulate and refine search strategy
- identify best source for specific information needs

If the general objectives for IM were broken down into specific objectives for each academic level they would be as follows:

By the end of the IM session, the first-year nursing student will:

1. be oriented to the physical arrangement of the library and library services provided.
2. be able to use the online catalog.
3. be aware of major nursing reference sources and major nursing textbooks.

The assignment for first-year nursing students is:

    a. use the online catalog to locate materials on a topic related to the course.
    b. use major reference sources and textbooks to define a topic relevant to the course.

A list of the sources consulted should be included with the worksheet.

By the end of the IM session, the second-year nursing student will:

1. be able to use CINAHL (printed and CD-ROM), and be aware of CINAHL online.
2. be able to use other nursing literature sources.

The assignment for second-year nursing students is:

    a. to identify appropriate subject headings using the CINAHL Subject Headings List, and
    b. to use the printed and CD-ROM versions to locate relevant information.

Topic for the assignment should be related to the course.

By the end of the IM session, the third-year nursing student will:

1. be able to use other indexing and abstracting services in the health sciences.
2. be able to use indexing and abstracting services and online systems in other disciplines.
3. be aware of citation indexing.

4. be able to formulate a search strategy (including dividing topic into concepts, using key words/free-text, using Boolean operators/proximity operators and using truncation), and be able to broaden or narrow a search.

An assignment created for this plan is to locate relevant information on a topic related to the course using appropriate indexes or databases.

By the end of the IM session, the fourth-year nursing student will:

1. be aware of current awareness strategies.
2. be aware of statistical sources.
3. be aware of Grateful MED.
4. be aware of electronic reprint management programs.
5. be aware of *Science Citation Index*, its concept and arrangement.
6. be able to identify the best source for specific information needs.
7. be aware of sources available using the Internet.

The assignment for fourth-year nursing students is to locate current articles on specific topics, locate statistics on specific topics, and identify the best place to look to answer specific patient-related questions. All questions should be related to the course.

Because nurses often attend graduate school a number of years after attending undergraduate school, it is important that a library orientation and a review of objectives should be given early in the graduate program. All of the objectives need to be covered, with the depth determined by the students' needs.

College of Allied Health Professionals

The general objectives for information management that were developed for the allied health students are listed below.[17,19-20]

An awareness of:

• physical arrangement of the library and library services provided
• methods of current awareness

- statistical sources
- Grateful MED
- reprint management programs
- citation indexing
- sources available using the Internet

The ability to:

- determine location of materials using an online catalog
- use major medical reference sources and textbooks
- use CINAHL (printed and CD-ROM)
- use *Index Medicus* and MEDLINE
- use indexing and abstracting services and online systems in the health sciences
- use indexing and abstracting services and online systems in other disciplines
- formulate and refine search strategy
- identify best source for specific information needs

At the University of South Alabama, all IM education for allied health students is covered during a required research class (junior level for one discipline and senior level for two disciplines). However, if IM for allied health students were included for the first through the fourth year at other institutions, the plan could contain the graduated objectives by level that follow.

By the end of the IM session, the first-year allied health student will:

1. be oriented to the physical arrangement of the library and the library services provided.
2. be able to use the online catalog.
3. be able to use major medical reference sources and textbooks.

An assignment for first-year allied health students is:

a. use the online catalog to locate materials on a topic related to the course.
b. use the major reference sources and textbooks to define a topic relevant to the course.

A list of the sources consulted should also be required.

By the end of the IM session, the second-year allied health student will:

1. be able to use CINAHL (printed and CD-ROM) and be aware of CINAHL online.
2. be able to access medical literature using other printed and electronic sources (*Index Medicus*, MEDLINE, etc.)

The assignment for second-year allied health students would be:
    a. identify appropriate subject headings using the CINAHL and MeSH subject headings lists.
    b. use the printed and CD-ROM versions of CINAHL and *Index Medicus*/MEDLINE to locate relevant information.

Topics should be related to the course.

By the end of the IM session, the third-year allied health student will:

1. be able to use other health science literature sources.
2. be able to use indexing and abstracting services and electronic systems in other disciplines.
3. be able to formulate a search strategy (including dividing topic into concepts, using keyword/free-text, using Boolean operators/proximity operators and using truncation) and be able to broaden or narrow a search.

An assignment created for this plan is to locate relevant information on a topic related to the course using appropriate indexes or databases.

By the end of the IM session, the fourth-year allied health student will:

1. be aware of current awareness strategies.
2. be aware of statistical sources.
3. be aware of Grateful MED.
4. be aware of electronic reprint management programs.
5. be aware of *Science Citation Index*, its concept and arrangement.

6. be aware of sources available using the Internet.
7. be able to identify the best source for specific information needs.

If divided into graduated objectives, the assignment for fourth-year allied health students could consist of locating current articles on specific topics, locating statistics on specific topics, and identifying the best place to look for answers to specific patient related questions. All questions should be related to the course.

As in nursing, graduate students in allied health should be given a general orientation to the library and the services provided, and instruction on use of the online catalog. All other objectives need to be covered, with the depth determined by the students' needs.

College of Medicine

"Physicians for the 21st Century: Report of the Project Panel on the General Professional Education of the Physician and College Preparation for Medicine" outlined five learning skills for medical students.[22] An IM program can contribute to three of the skills:

1. retrieve valid and relevant information on a patient care question from an institutional library; use computerized information retrieval systems.
2. develop and use a personal filing system for storing and retrieving relevant information.
3. become familiar with a range of professional journals and texts and develop an efficient browsing strategy where decisions are rapidly made about which articles are valid and applicable.

For the College of Medicine students, the following general objectives of information management were developed.[11,15,17,20,23-26] An awareness of:

- the physical arrangement of the library and library services provided
- NLM classification system
- indexing specificity rule

- various software programs and database vendors used for on-line searching
- statistical sources
- methods of current awareness
- reprint management programs
- citation indexing
- sources available using the Internet

The ability to:

- determine the location of materials using an online catalog
- use basic medical reference sources and textbooks
- use *Index Medicus* and MEDLINE to retrieve relevant information
- use indexing and abstracting services and online systems in the health sciences
- use indexing and abstracting services and online systems in other disciplines
- formulate and refine a search strategy
- use Grateful MED
- identify the best sources for specific information needs
- access medical literature when outside a medical center environment

As with nursing and allied health students, IM for medical students should be a building process and can be taught using a problem based format.[15] Below are the objectives by academic level.

The objective of information management for first-year medical students is to orient students to the basic organization of the library, to introduce the core basic medical science monographic and journal literature, and to provide an overview to *Index Medicus* and MEDLINE.

By the end of the IM session, the first-year medical student will:

1. be oriented to the physical arrangement of the library and be aware of library services provided.
2. be able to use the online catalog.
3. be aware of the NLM classification scheme.
4. be aware of medical reference sources and the standard basic medical science textbooks.

5. be able to use *Index Medicus*, including MeSH headings and subheadings, tree structure, and Bibliography of Medical Reviews and be aware of the history and scope of *Index Medicus*/MEDLINE.
6. understand the indexing specificity rule.
7. be familiar with the *List of Journals Indexed in Index Medicus*.
8. be able to use MEDLINE on CD-ROM.

The assignment for first-year medical students is:

a. to identify sources that define and describe a syndrome.
b. identify the correct MeSH headings and subheadings and indicate how it is arranged in the tree structure.
c. locate review articles on the syndrome.
d. use the online catalog to obtain book titles on the syndrome.

A list of sources consulted by the student, and a printout of the OPAC screen should be part of the assignment. A specific patient management question should be used, and the assignment should be course-related.

By the end of the IM session, the second-year medical student will:

1. be familiar with the use of MeSH terms and subheadings, and the tree structure.
2. be able to use the CD-ROM system for MEDLINE.
3. be able to formulate and refine search strategy (including dividing the search topic into concepts, using keyword/free-text in searching, using Boolean operators and proximity operators, and using truncation in searching) and be able to broaden or narrow a search strategy.
4. be able to use other indexing and abstracting services and online systems in the health sciences.
5. be able to use *Science Citation Index*, and be aware of its concept and arrangement.
6. be aware of indexing and abstracting services and online systems in other disciplines.
7. be able to retrieve research article on a clinical subject.

The assignment for second-year medical students is to:

>   a. turn in a printout of a search that they performed on a topic related to the course using the CD-ROM system.
>   b. obtain relevant articles from *SCI* using the Permuterm and/ or *Citation Index*.

By the end of the IM session, the third-year medical student will:

1. be aware of the basic texts and journals in clinical medicine.
2. be familiar with the use of *Index Medicus* (MeSH and sub-headings, and tree structure).
3. be familiar with the use of MEDLINE.
4. be able to use Grateful MED.
5. be aware of BRS Colleague and other end-user search systems.
6. be aware of methods of current awareness.
7. be aware of reprint management methods.
8. be aware of sources available using the Internet.
9. be able to identify the best sources for specific information needs.
10. be aware of methods used to access medical information outside a medical environment.

The assignment for third-year medical students is to use Grateful MED and the CD-ROM system to locate citations relevant to a patient management question.

Discussion of *Index Medicus*/MEDLINE and CINAHL is a very important aspect of the IM plan. By the end of the presentation on *Index Medicus*/MEDLINE and/or CINAHL, the student will:

1. understand the scope and history of the index and/or database.
2. be able to use the thesaurus (MeSH and CINAHL subject headings–annotated alphabetical, permuted, and tree structure) to determine relevant subject headings, including "see references."
3. be able to use the Author and Subject sections of printed indexes, understand the meaning of a title in brackets in *Index*

Medicus/MEDLINE, and be able to identify the components of a citation.

4. be able to use the Bibliography of Medical Reviews in *Index Medicus* to retrieve review articles and be able to retrieve review articles on MEDLINE and/or CINAHL (online or CD-ROM).
5. be able to use the *List of Journal Indexed in Index Medicus* and "Journals and Serials Indexed" in CINAHL.
6. be able to use subheadings and check tags.
7. be able to divide a search topic into concepts.
8. be able to use Boolean operators and proximity operators.
9. be able to narrow or broaden a search in a CD-ROM or online search.
10. be able to use keywords and free-text searching in CD-ROM or online search and be aware of when such use is appropriate.
11. be able to use truncation in CD-ROM or online search.
12. be able to use explosions in CD-ROM or online search.

DISCUSSION

A teaching plan, such as this plan for information management instruction, is never completed. It requires constant revision in order to incorporate new technology, changing curricula, and the varying needs of the students. Communication channels between the library faculty and the faculty in each college must be kept open. This project has helped to assure that information management will not be a haphazard event where library instruction is often either repetitive or lacking. Written objectives for each course help the library faculty eliminate gaps and overlap in library instruction for the students. Establishment of this plan has also helped to enhance the image of the librarians by giving them a more visible and viable role in the design of the curriculum for each of the colleges.

The following suggestions should prove helpful when trying to integrate an information management plan into the curriculum:

- *Have a vision.* Determine the direction that information management instruction needs to take at your institution.

- *Have a plan with detailed objectives.* Because educators work with objectives, they deal best with specific objectives rather than with lengthy text.
- *Be brief.* Be willing to work with the busy schedules of administrators and do not take any more time than is absolutely necessary.
- *Listen to suggestions.* Librarians know best what information management skills the students should learn. Professors in the disciplines know best how those skills fit into the overall curriculum plan.
- *Be patient.* Working within the academic system, this plan took about a year from development to implementation. In the world of academics, one learns to be patient.
- *Make allies.* Promote the plan during all opportunities. While those listening may not have the final voice in making decisions, they can be supporters when the plan is presented.
- *Enjoy the process.* In addition to making a contribution to the information management skills of the students with whom they work, the library faculty is also being established as authorities with the faculty in those departments.

REFERENCES

1. Rader, H., and Coons, W. "Information Literacy: One Response to the New Decade." In: *The Evolving Educational Mission of the Library*, edited by Baker, B., and Litzinger, M.E. Chicago: Association of College and Research Libraries, 1992, pp. 109-127.

2. Haskell, D.A. "The Role of the Clinical Medical Librarian in Medical Education." *Clinical Librarian Quarterly* 2(4, 1984):6-9.

3. Reidelbach, M.A.; Willis, D.B.; Kinecky, J.L.; Rasmussen, R.J.; and Stark, J. "An Introduction to Independent Learning Skills for Incoming Medical Students." *Bulletin of the Medical Library Association* 76(April 1988):159-163.

4. Burrows, S.; Ginn, D.S.; Love, N.; and Williams, T.L. "A Strategy for Curriculum Integration of Information Skills Instruction." *Bulletin of the Medical Library Association* 77(July 1989):245-251.

5. "State-of-the-Art in Medical Informatics." *Journal of Medical Education* 61(June 1986):489-543.

6. Allegri, F. "Course Integrated Instruction: Metamorphosis for the Twenty-First Century." *Medical Reference Services Quarterly* 4(Winter 1985/86):47-66.

7. Kimmel, S. "Teaching Third-Year Medical Students to Search MEDLINE." *Medical Reference Services Quarterly* 8(Fall 1989):69-76

8. Martin, J.A. "Bibliographic Instruction in the Medical Library." *Tennessee Librarian* (Spring 1980):10-12.

9. Fick, G.R. "Integrating Bibliographic Instruction into an Undergraduate Nursing Curriculum." *Bulletin of the Medical Library Association* 76(July 1988): 269-271.

10. Gondek, V.A. and Romanos, V.M. "A Basic Program of Bibliographic Instruction in a Health Sciences Library." *Medical Reference Services Quarterly* 2(Fall 1983):83-89.

11. Loftin, J.E. "Library Orientation and Library Instruction for Medical Students." *Bulletin of the Medical Library Association* 71(April 1983):207-209.

12. Tyler, J.K., and Switzer, J.H. "Meeting the Information Needs of Nursing Students: A Library Instruction Module for a Nursing Research Class." *Medical Reference Services Quarterly* 10(Fall 1991):39-44.

13. Iroka, L.A. "Library Orientation and Instruction for Medical Students." *International Library Review* 21 (1989):481-485.

14. Carroad, E.G., and McGregor, G. "Teaching Role of the Health Science Library" in *Handbook of Medical Library Practice*, 4th edition. Edited by L. Darling. Chicago: Medical Library Association, 1982, p. 237-271.

15. Dorsch, J.L.; Frasca, M.A.; Wilson, M.L.; and Tomsic, M.L. "A Multidisciplinary Approach to Information and Critical Appraisal Instruction." *Bulletin of the Medical Library Association* 78 (January 1990):38-44.

16. Graves, K.J. "Bibliographic Instruction for Graduate Students in the Health Sciences." *Medical Reference Services Quarterly* 1(Fall 1982):73-81.

17. Winiarz, E., and Sullivan, S.J. "Discovering the Variety of Library Resources through Bibliographic Instruction and an Assignment." *Canadian Library Journal* 48 (October 1991):335-338.

18. Walser, K.P., and Kruse, K.W. "A College Course for Nurses on the Utilization of Library Resources." *Bulletin of the Medical Library Association* 65(April 1977):265-267.

19. Branch, K. "Developing a Conceptual Framework for Teaching End-User Searching." *Medical Reference Services Quarterly* 5(Spring 1986):71-76.

20. Port, J., and Meiss, H.R. "Teaching Library Skills to Third-Year Clerkships." *Journal of Medical Education* 57(July 1982):564-566.

21. Tucker, D.C., and Giger, J.N. *Finding Nursing (in the Library): A Student Manual of Information Retrieval and Utilization Skills*. Bristol, IN: Wyndham Hall Press, 1990.

22. "Physicians for the 21st Century: Report on the Project Panel on the General Professional Education of the Physician and College Preparation for Medicine." *Journal of Medical Education* 59(November 1984):1-159.

23. Allen, S.N.; Mahan, J.M.; and Graham, I. "The Implementation of a Large-Scale Self-Instructional Course in Medical Information Resources." *Bulletin of the Medical Library Association* 67(July 1979):302-307.

24. Graves, K.J., and Selig, S.A. "Library Instruction for Medical Students." *Bulletin of the Medical Library Association* 74(April 1986):126-130.

25. Mueller, M.H., and Foreman, G. "Library Instruction for Medical Students During Curriculum Elective." *Bulletin of the Medical Library Association* 75(July 1987):253-256.

26. Whitsed, N. "CD-ROM: An End-User Training Tool?–The Experience of Using Medline in a Small Medical School Library." *Program* 23(April 1989): 117-126.

27. Frasca, M.A.; Dorsch, J.L.; Aldag, J.C.; and Christiansen, R.G. "A Multi-disciplinary Approach to Information Management and Critical Appraisal Instruction: A Controlled Study." *Bulletin of the Medical Library Association* 80(January 1992):23-28.

PART V

COMPUTER-ASSISTED INSTRUCTION AND AUDIOVISUAL AIDS

Chapter 25

Library Orientation on Videotape: Production Planning and Administrative Support

James Shedlock
Edward W. Tawyea

INTRODUCTION

Northwestern University Medical Library (NUML) has continued to develop its media production capabilities since 1983. In 1986, it began installation of video production and viewing facilities to take advantage of new technologies and to meet the demands of Northwestern users. The facility includes photography, video production, and computer graphics services.

The media production facility is housed in laboratory space within the Medical School and consists of the following hardware configuration: JVC three-gun color video cameras; JVC video switcher; Tascam audio mixer; Sony three-machine editing configuration; Nova time-base correctors; Grass Valley master synch generator; and Lumena 16 graphics software operating on an IBM AT with an AT&T Targa 16 graphics board and a Kurta digitizing tablet. This configuration allows the media production staff to mix and edit audio, video, and computer-generated images. The graphics software provides for the conversion of full-color video images to full-color digitized computer images.

This chapter was originally presented at the 1987 annual meeting of the Medical Library Association in Portland, OR. This chapter was first published in *Medical Reference Services Quarterly*, Vol. 8(2), Summer 1989.

The availability of the new video production unit provides other public services the opportunity to utilize media in service applications. At Northwestern, reference staff needed a new way to orient first-year medical students and other health sciences students to the library and its services because group walking tours finally proved unsatisfactory. The expanded media production unit allowed reference staff to put the orientation tour on videotape.

LITERATURE REVIEW

While the published literature is not extensive, it does show that some librarians are using various media and new technologies to improve and enhance library instruction and orientation. In an early report, Key and Tollman[1] describe a library instruction videotape at the University of Nebraska aimed at undergraduate students. Their report indicates how librarians worked with the campus TV station staff to produce the videotape. Their purpose was similar to the Northwestern need: "to find a more efficient way to provide library instruction.'" Kautz, Rodkewich, and Philipson describe the use of interactive video for library instruction at the University of Minnesota.[2] Microcomputer programs control the videotape to effect a structured lesson that includes text and live action. Besides instruction, videotape can be used in library training sessions. Crawford describes using videotape to teach new student employees how to perform circulation tasks.[3]

The lack of a video production unit within the library, however, should not deter public service departments from considering video projects. Reference librarians and other public service staff can consider working with video units from the medical school, hospital, or university on an intra-institutional cooperative basis similar to the arrangement described by Key and Tollman. For example, Brassil in 1983 utilized other university departments at the University of North Carolina at Chapel Hill to produce an orientation videotape for the Health Sciences Library.[4] This videotape became the model for the Northwestern project. In 1985 White produced a videotape that describes and highlights the services of area health education center (AHEC) libraries.[5] In 1986 Allegri revised the 1983 North Carolina orientation tape and highlighted services without stressing a walk-through tour; a special feature of the revised tape is its utilization of staff interviews to describe library services.[6]

BACKGROUND

The proximity of a video production unit within the library is an advantage for NUML reference staff. Communication is easier and contact with members of the two departments is frequent; staff know how to work with each other and recognize mutual service goals.

Library orientation was considered for videotaping for a number of reasons. Like most older library buildings, Northwestern's Medical Library makes it awkward to tour large groups of users and introduce them to the collection and library services. The videotape can act as a guide through the library and reinforce messages about building use that are likely to get lost in a tour. Orientation for the freshman class of 170 students was a particular problem. Group tours of the library, with some added emphasis on services and instruction, was the old model; the videotape concept allows a library tour and instruction for 170 students at one time.

Northwestern librarians quickly realized the advantages of using videotape to deliver valuable instructional messages to users and decided to incorporate tips on how to use the library for research purposes. The project concept included not just the physical tour of the library and an introduction to its services (circulation services and library cards, photocopy access, etc.), but also covered such topics as: using *Medical Subject Headings*; using LUIS, the Library User Information Service, Northwestern's online public access catalog; how to use subject headings to search in LUIS; what is an index and how to use *Index Medicus*; and how to plan a search strategy that satisfies an information need. The videotape would consist of two sections conveying important information about the library as a service center and as a resource. Both sections were accommodated in a 15-minute tape.

A common theme highlighted in the cited literature was again verified by the Northwestern project, namely, the need to conserve staff energy during the orientation season and to improve library instruction methods with some "pizazz." Having one solid presentation also improves consistency in the messages delivered to new library users; the videotape concept is ideal in achieving this goal.

Because the videotape is portable, staff can disseminate information about the library to remote groups and bring the library to them. The Northwestern tape also served another purpose by "showing off" the media production capabilities within the library.

PLANNING PROCESS

Planning is the most important aspect of producing a videotape. The more thought and decision making that can be done in advance, the more likely a quality product will result from the effort. Using the orientation tape as a model, the first step in the planning process is to outline a preliminary schedule.

A schedule is necessary to keep the project on a firm timetable. Knowing when the videotape is to be used for its debut is an important incentive in completing the project. Scheduling helps keep the project moving and prevents it from bogging down or being distracted by other service needs. At Northwestern, the videotape was needed for freshman orientation in September 1986, so planning began in early summer with taping scheduled for late July and early August.

An outline of goals is the second planning step. The librarian-director must define the purpose and focus of the tape as well as its intended audience. At Northwestern, the goal was to orient freshmen students and any new faculty or staff to the Medical Library. A secondary goal was to instruct the viewer on how to use the library to his/her advantage. Without defined goals, the focus of the tape becomes confused and production becomes difficult.

Drafting the script is the third planning step. The draft should be informative but also must adhere strictly to the goals outlined for the project. The draft for an orientation tape should contain as much information as possible; editing will eliminate minor points as well as nonessential material. The draft should be reviewed by as many readers as possible to get their ideas and to check if the videotape is meeting staff expectations.

The next step is to identify the visual scenes that will accompany the script. This outline should include brief notations on how the librarian-director views the parts of the script along with any ideas for visualizing the script. One good way to do this is to print the script in a two-column format, with the script in the right-side column and space for notations in the left-side column. Creative ideas that enhance the visuals should be noted. The script should be examined for concepts that are especially difficult to represent in a visual way, and efforts should be made to concentrate on these shots. Another tip is to be conscious of time. It takes far less time to do an activity than it takes the narrator to describe the same activity in words. The visual scenes should be planned so that the activity takes the same amount of time as it takes to describe the activity orally.

Another important step is to do storyboards. Storyboards are pictorial sketches of a scene and its accompanying dialogue. Storyboards allow the scriptwriter to map the script to a visual scene. This process forces the producers to make sure each sentence of the script is visually represented on the videotape. Without the storyboards, the script is likely to get away from its visual counterpart, and some information will be left with blank tape to represent it. Storyboards play an essential role in the planning process and communicate to the video cameraman what he should look for in a visual scene.

The culmination of the planning effort is the actual shooting of scenes. Planning is also important here because it takes away the element of surprise from staff, alerts all library staff to prepare for the taping, and elicits cooperation from everyone involved. Scheduling here is also important so staff know when they may be on camera; scheduling also helps identify staff members who are extremely camera-shy. If library staff will appear on camera without speaking parts, they should be instructed as to what to do and what to wear. Color visuals are most important in a videotape and light-colored clothing produces a poorer image. At Northwestern, the orientation tape used a minimum of acting for demonstrating services. Depending on local resources and budgets, actors may be used for this type of videotape. Local talent should be considered from among the library staff, campus drama departments, or local amateur theater groups. Using actors may not require monetary compensation for individuals seeking experience in this type of production. Offers of a free copy of the finished videotape may be all that is required for payment.

Another important point in shooting scenes is to take as many extra shots as possible. Like script writing, having extra footage offers a selection of scenes to incorporate into the tape. Editing also eliminates the poor quality material. Still another point is to plan the camera work so that shooting in the same area takes place at the same time since moving camera equipment and camera set-up takes time and effort.

Editing completes the production process by bringing together all the parts of the videotape and prepares the final product. Editing is time-consuming. A general rule to remember is that two hours of editing is needed to complete one minute of tape. While editing is the longest segment of production for a neophyte, it becomes the most exciting part. In editing, the video expert shows his/her professional skill, and the librarian-director has an opportunity to be involved in the creative process of combining, splicing, and dubbing footage, decisions that determine the final product. The editing process includes decisions on the best sequence of shots to represent the script, what slides to use to mix with live action, what music to use for introduction and closing scenes, who will read the script for the narration, and what text to use for instructional components. At Northwestern, all the editing took place in-house except for the narration, which involved a graduate student from the School of Journalism and used the School of Medicine's Hearing Clinics for taping in their sound-proof rooms.

The final step in planning and production is the preliminary showing to, and evaluation by, library staff. Once fully edited, very little change can be made to a videotape since all the elements–narration, visuals, and text–are synchronized. The most that the evaluation can do is teach the producers how to prepare for the second edition of the tape.

ADMINISTRATIVE SUPPORT
AND COST ANALYSIS

From an administrative standpoint, the production of this videotape meant the allocation of significant resources over several months' time. Since the library controlled all of the means of production, very little money was exchanged for this project. For illustrative purposes, a simple cost breakdown is provided. Costs are in terms of the staff time spent on the entire project and the cost of utilizing the taping and editing facilities (based on the hourly charges for these facilities as set by the library).

Time of Video Technician

Videotaping	=	40 Hrs
Editing	=	49 Hrs
TOTAL	=	89 Hrs

Time of Video Production Assistant

Videotaping	=	40 Hrs
Photography	=	6 Hrs
TOTAL	=	46 Hrs

Time of Head of Public Services

Script Writing	=	15 Hrs
Videotaping	=	40 Hrs
Editing	=	40 Hrs
TOTAL	=	95 Hrs

Time of Narrator

Script Reading = 3 Hrs

Based upon the hourly wages and fringe benefits for these staff members, the total labor costs are estimated at $3,732. All wages are calculated per 1986, the year the tape was produced.

The cost of utilizing Northwestern's editing facilities is $980. Material costs (videotape, slides, etc.) were $131. The total cost of this production was $4,843. The estimate for having this same tape produced by a private firm is $8,400. It should be noted, however, that video production costs have been lower elsewhere.[7]

Analyzing the benefit of the tape in relation to its cost is extremely difficult. Initially, the calculation was done on the basis of the number of hours the tape would be utilized by individuals. The rationale for the calculation was that if the tape was viewed by users, it would reduce the time reference staff needed to spend on individual orientations. Time savings are for group orientations not factored in the cost-benefit analysis since reference staff are needed in group presentations to answer questions after the video is shown. Unfortunately, the tape has been lightly used by individuals outside of orientation sessions.

Existing data on use to date confirms that the cost of producing this videotape is not justified utilizing the simple cost-benefit analysis above. The public service librarians believe, however, that this project is still worthwhile and that ultimately the benefits outweigh the costs involved. These benefits include a reduction in the amount of time reference staff are involved in the repetitious task of teaching new users about library services and facilities, having the orientation tape available at times when a reference staff member is not available such as late evenings and Sundays, and taking the tape into areas of the medical center in which staff have no knowledge of the library at all. In this way the tape also serves as a marketing tool for the library.

DISCUSSION

The primary benefit of the tape appears to be in providing a stimulating and consistent orientation to the library and its services. The tape gives libraries and librarians a very positive image. It also relieves the reference staff of the task of repeating the same information during orientations and frees them to respond to questions or to present specialized information for the selected group.

Whether the same information could be communicated better and more inexpensively with other technology is still in question. A slide presentation would allow the library to update the program regularly since it provides discrete information and images. It lacks, however, the continuity of motion which is useful in demonstrating certain activities, e.g., online searching. A very interesting option to video would be the use of desktop presentation software. This technology allows for the presentation of "live" computerized images, including animation and digitized color photographs. It also has the advantage of being easily updated without the necessity of utilizing expensive video equipment and editing facilities. Hypermedia may also provide more options for conveying instructional messages to users.

CONCLUSION

There are still many questions left unanswered regarding video for library instruction: do users prefer videotape instruction to live sessions; do users learn better with video than in live sessions; does video orientation reduce the number of directional questions users are likely to ask?

The initial trial with video orientation has been encouraging. On the basis of this experience, Northwestern librarians are considering the production of a tape to orient new staff members to the circulation department and the NOTIS online circulation system. This is another area in which the amount of time staff spend in repetitious orientations can be reduced. Video remains a powerful tool in educating users and staff.

REFERENCES

1. Key, Janet, and Tollman, Thomas A. *Videotape as an Aid to Bibliographic Instruction.* 1981. ERIC document ED206319.

2. Kautz, Barbara A.; Rodkewich, Patricia M.; and Philipson, Will D. "The Evolution of a New Library Instruction Concept: Interactive Video (at the University of Minnesota, Minneapolis-St. Paul)." *Research Strategies* 6(Summer 1988): 109-117.

3. Crawford, Gregory A. "Training Student Employees by Videotape." *College & Research Libraries News* 49(March 1988):149-150,152.

4. Brassil, Ellen Christine. *Introduction to the Health Sciences Library.* Chapel Hill, North Carolina: Health Sciences Library, University of North Carolina at Chapel Hill, 1983.

5. White, Cathryn E. *Information Services for Dental Professionals.* Chapel Hill, North Carolina: Health Sciences Library, University of North Carolina at Chapel Hill, 1985.

6. Allegri, Francesca. *Health Sciences Library Orientation.* Chapel Hill, North Carolina: Health Sciences Library, University of North Carolina at Chapel Hill, 1986.

7. Smith, Jean. "Teaching Research Skills Using Video: An Undergraduate Approach." *Reference Services Review* 16(1-2, 1988):109-114.

Chapter 26

Watch Your Language:
A CAI Approach to Teaching MeSH

Nancy Calabretta
Elizabeth Mikita
Elizabeth Warner
Joyce Bryant
Margaret Devlin
Barbara Laynor

Computer applications in libraries have focused on automating internal library functions, designing online public catalogs, and accessing remote or CD-ROM databases. Once computers have become a part of the daily library routine, it is logical to explore other ways to apply the technology. The Association of Academic Health Sciences Library Directors report, *Challenge to Action: Planning and Evaluation Guidelines for Academic Health Science Libraries,* states:

> The Library should be instrumental in the institution's plan to integrate computing and non-print learning resources into the curriculum; it also must assume a broader role in assisting students, faculty, and practitioners to master basic skills in information handling.[1]

In many libraries, this "broader role" has translated into a rapid expansion of user education programs. At the same time, authoring

This chapter was first published in *Medical Reference Services Quarterly,* Vol. 9(4), Winter 1990.

packages and hypermedia, which promise to eliminate the need for professional programmers, have regenerated interest in computer-assisted instruction (CAI) software as a teaching tool.

The use of computer-assisted instruction in biomedical education began in the early 1960s, but declined during the 1970s. Early CAI programs ran on large, expensive mainframe computers, accessible over telephone lines, with the capacity for timesharing. An instructor who wanted to develop a CAI tool needed not only subject expertise but also experience in instructional design and programming. In the 1980s, CAI programs are more commonly run on less expensive, easy-to-use microcomputers, now an essential component of most educational settings. The most successful health science developers have focused on the computer's potential for interactive, individualized instruction to create simulations of clinical encounters. As Piemme stated in a comprehensive review of CAI, "computer technology has the power and the capacity to facilitate independent learning and to teach problem solving in a manner unmatched by any other medium."[2] Presented with an opportunity to apply for grant monies to support a CAI development project, library staff at Scott Memorial Library (SML), Thomas Jefferson University, posed the following questions: Could CAI be useful for user education programs? Would it be worthwhile for librarians to produce CAI programs for this purpose?

HEALTH SCIENCES LIBRARIES CONSORTIUM GRANTS

In 1988, the Health Sciences Libraries Consortium (HSLC),[3] in conjunction with the Philadelphia Liaison Committee on Computers in Medical Education, established a grant program to help fund development of computer-assisted instruction at member institutions. Specifically, HSLC sought to encourage creation of original programs and implementation of CAI to promote self-directed learning among students, improve skills and habits necessary for lifelong learning, and foster innovation in teaching among faculty and staff of the member institutions. While targeted mainly at faculty and students, staff members of HSLC institutions were also eligible to apply for these grants. The objective was to create a collection of programs to be shared by HSLC members.

What library/information skills topic could be selected which had widest applicability to learning needs across all HSLC institutions and beyond? A large multisite audience required a topic which was not system-specific, which could be used by all HSLC members, and which was relevant to health care practitioners as well as students. Because it is used universally in health sciences libraries by all health sciences disciplines, Medical Subject Headings (MeSH) seemed an appropriate topic for this new learning tool. SML staff submitted a grant proposal for a CAI, program titled *Watch Your Language: MeSH and the Health Sciences Literature User,* to enhance the SML user education program as well as serve the training needs of the other HSLC institutions. The project was viewed as an opportunity to produce a useful program while increasing computer skills and knowledge about alternative instructional methods.

An authoring package had to be specified and justified in the grant application. Because SML is a Macintosh microcomputer environment, the selection process centered on Mac-based authoring systems. The Director of the Office of Academic Computing had viewed a pre-release version of Authorware's *Course of Action*™ (now known as Authorware Academic)[4] and was impressed with its ease of use. An Apple computer comparison of Macintosh authoring software emphasized that *Course of Action*™ is a visual icon-based authoring system designed especially for people who have no knowledge of programming."[5] Designed by educators specifically for CAI, *Course of Action*™ also provided "portability"–a program built on the Macintosh could be converted to IBM format in the future. This was felt to further enhance the final product's usefulness outside SML.

The grant application was successful and $5,038 was awarded in April 1988. Of 24 CAI proposals funded by the Health Sciences Libraries Consortium for the 1988-89 project year, the Scott Memorial Library project was the only one designed to teach library/information skills. Grant funds subsidized the purchase of a Macintosh SE and authoring software. The funds also covered the services of a consultant from Thomas Jefferson University's Office of Academic Computing and payment for student evaluators of the program. The grant requirements stipulated that "faculty" (i.e., staff) time must be donated. A six-member Task Force of SML staff was formed, and the project was completed in less than four months. This chapter describes: (1) the process used in completing the project; (2) the feasibility of in-house CAI production for library user education; and (3) the appropriateness of CAI instruction for teaching MeSH.

MeSH

The *Medical Subject Headings* (MeSH) thesaurus can be seen as both the major aid and the major obstacle to effective searching of the health sciences literature. Familiarity with MeSH cross-references, subheadings, and tree structures is crucial to health sciences library users everywhere. Yet, providing even a basic level of training for a broad range of users has proven time-consuming and labor-intensive for many libraries. Many library users have encountered and used controlled vocabularies. Most, however, have not considered why they could not find the subject heading they thought should exist. Why, for example, should they have to search CEREBROVASCULAR DISORDERS for information on strokes? The fact that the tree structures impose a hierarchical structure with lengthy alphanumeric character strings on the MeSH vocabulary often complicates rather then clarifies the thesaurus for users. Further contributing to the complexity of MeSH are factors such as inverted headings, precoordinated headings, specialty headings, "general only" headings, and generic drug names. SML staff concluded that there was a real need for a self-guided MeSH teaching tool that: (1) could be used either individually or in small groups; (2) would be available at the point of need, rather than in a classroom setting; and (3) would cover basic concepts and not be tied to a specific annual edition of *MeSH.*

TEAM APPROACH

Even though current authoring software is easier and more user-friendly than previous generations, a great deal of time is required to produce a finished product. A team approach seemed practical and efficient for this project. A six-member Task Force was formed–one team of three to write the script and another team of three to work with the authoring system. As the Script Team wrote and rewrote, the design team concentrated on a "quick learn" of the software. Procedures were established by the Task Force that required the Script Team and the Design Team to refer draft products to each other. Often, especially in the beginning, the text had to be streamlined so that there were fewer words per screen and more room for graphics. The resulting screens were then reviewed by the Script Team to ensure that the intended information was clearly conveyed. While the team division was necessary from a practical perspective, each Task Force member was encouraged to be flexible. The Script Team could suggest graphics and gimmicks to the Design Team which could, in turn, suggest script ideas or changes. Some attempts were immediately successful; others were not. However, the interactive process allowed the two teams to make the fullest use of the talents of each member.

Script Team

Members of the Script Team–all with experience in teaching MeSH in a variety of situations to a variety of users–came to the project with an interesting collection of materials, lectures, and exercises that had been developed for MeSH instruction. Most of these proved to be inappropriate for the CAI format which requires, above all, concise wording and graphic images. A new style of writing, different from that used for a formal paper yet unlike that of an oral presentation, was required. It was felt that most users were unfamiliar with the theoretical background that librarians have and would, therefore, benefit from a limited introduction to controlled vocabularies and to the basics of MeSH. They would not want, or need, to know everything about MeSH. The goal was to reach a wide range of users at an introductory level. To keep themselves on track, the Script Team compiled the following set of guidelines to consider as they wrote:

- Think users–not librarians.
- Think rules–not expectations.
- Think graphics.
- Think action.

- Think tone (engaging–fun, but not silly).
- Length of explanation = importance of point.

An early, but controversial, Script Team decision to use the "Black and White" *MeSH* as the source of examples and illustrations helped to maintain the focus on basics. In most libraries, "Black and White" *MeSH* is the tool made available to the public and, unlike *Medical Subject Headings–Annotated Alphabetic List (Annotated MeSH)*, it is primarily designed for the end user. There are fewer and less complex annotations, and the difference between "major" and "minor" headings is much clearer than in *Annotated MeSH.*

The Script Team chose to create brief modules followed by summaries designed to reinforce information. Each module covered a specific concept and built on earlier modules. The introductory modules covered basic concepts such as controlled vocabulary, cross-references, and the *Tree Structures.* Separate modules were devoted to the application of MeSH beyond *Index Medicus,* so that users would understand how MeSH could be applied differently in other bibliographic resources such as computer-based systems and library catalogs. A final module was designed for allied health professionals, covering the use and enhancement of MeSH in *Cumulative Index to Nursing and Allied Health Literature (CINAHL).*

Design Team

Familiarity with other Macintosh applications enabled the Design Team to begin creating a simple program with little preparation or practice. The structure and capabilities of *Course of Action* software guided the designers. The basic functions of the software are controlled by icons–pictorial representations of the software's specific capabilities (see Figure 26.1). For example, an eraser icon is used to erase. Using the software's drawing tools, the Design Team created original drawings and imported illustrations from other sources. These illustrations–and text as well–could appear and disappear in a variety of ways, such as fading in and out or moving across the screen at different speeds.

The Design Team experimented with the software while working with early script drafts. Initial successes and failures were shared

FIGURE 26.1. Course of Action™ ICONS

⬜	Display Icon	Text and graphics in course presentation window
	Animation Icon	Selection of display to be animated, movement options
	Erase Icon	Selection of display to be erased, effects options
(WAIT)	Wait Icon	Prompting and timing options
◇	Decision Icon	Path selection, repetition, and time limit options
⟨?⟩	Question Icon	Answer-evaluation options, character limit, and question erasure; pushbutton to edit the Question display
▣	Calculation Icon	Window for calculation and assignments, calls to user-written code, and jumps to other applications
🗺	Map Icon	A course flow line window

with the entire Task Force to encourage realistic expectations. For example, a screen display which would simulate the turning of pages was suggested, but the actualization of this idea was too time-consuming and complicated for the Design Team to produce using the current version of the software. After examining several CAI products and surveying the literature on CAI production (see Appendix), the Design Team developed guidelines for creating *Watch Your Language:*

1. Use one typeface. A simple font called New York was selected to be used throughout the program.
2. Locate all return "buttons" in the lower right hand corner of each screen.
3. Limit use of animation and illustrations to the examples so as not to detract from factual information.
4. Provide variety by creating distinctive backgrounds for each module.
5. Include online instructions and pull-down menus to provide user assistance.
6. Allow users to change screens or quit the program at any time.

By following these guidelines, the Design Team established consistency within the program. Users can recognize where they are and move easily through the program. Changing patterns and displays add interest to the screens, while the consistent presentation of information–text in one area of the screen, illustrations in another–helps reinforce learning.

As the project progressed, the Script Team refined its objectives and simplified the script to conform to the concept of an introductory MeSH program. The Design Team became adept at breaking the text into screens while maintaining the integrity of the script. The program went through dozens of rewrites and screen changes as the Design Team learned to use the advanced features of the software to accomplish more of what the Script Team visualized. After much interaction, each team gave final approval to a module and moved on to the next module. When the program was complete, each Task Force member reviewed it screen by screen to ensure consistency and accuracy. Everyone involved in the project gave their stamp of approval to the final product.

THE PROJECT

The final product, titled *Watch Your Language Version 1.0*, consists of nine content modules, a pretest, and a posttest. The nine content modules introduce and describe MeSH; its purpose; its arrangement; rules for use in *Index Medicus*, MEDLINE, and library catalogs; and the MeSH-based *Nursing and Allied Health*

Subject Heading List. Brief "tip" screens highlight key concepts. Each module concludes with one screen which summarizes that module's content (see Figure 26.2). The program begins with a short pretest and ends with a posttest. Graphics and examples are used throughout (see Figure 26.3). The product itself fits onto a single disk; viewing time runs approximately 45 minutes.

EVALUATION

Preliminary evaluation consisted of a field test by nine paid volunteers. The evaluators included one medical student, one life sciences student, two college graduates without health care backgrounds (to simulate incoming students), and two library school students. Evaluators were asked to note their comments on a form provided, or to provide oral comments during the use of the program. A member of the Task Force observed and interviewed each evaluator. The overall rating was positive, with the most enthusiastic reviews coming from the library school students. Speed of the program, the sequence of some screens, and several examples were changed after this initial evaluation.

PRODUCT PROMOTION

Since completing the program, the six Task Force members have been investigating methods for marketing and distribution. At Scott Memorial Library the first step was to place a Macintosh SE with a copy of *Watch Your Language* adjacent to the Information Desk. Since this is where users encounter tools such as miniMEDLINE, CD Plus MEDLINE, and standard print indexes, staff will be able to introduce the program at the point of need. Copies have also been placed in the Library's Learning Resources Center to accommodate individual viewing. In addition, the User Education staff plans to integrate the program into its workshop and classes. It is too soon to assess the effectiveness of these efforts.

End users showed a great deal of interest in *Watch Your Language* when it was demonstrated at a local Macintosh "Computers

FIGURE 26.2. Summary Screen Example

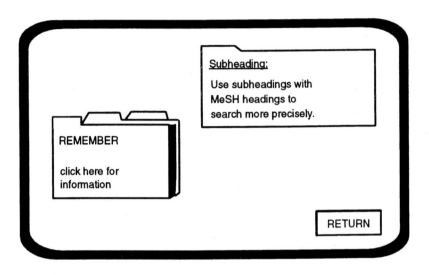

FIGURE 26.3. Tree Structure Graphic

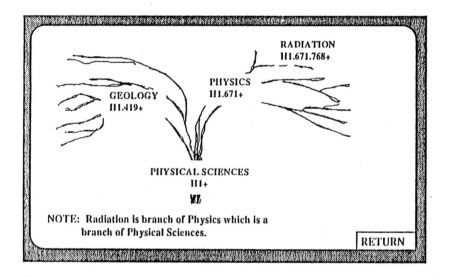

in Medicine" conference. Several physicians have requested copies for their own use. Thus, practicing health care professionals who search MEDLINE from home or office appear to be a good target audience. By offering the program to other libraries as shareware, users in other institutions may benefit from this CAI development effort. In time, the Task Force plans to survey both librarians and end users to assess the effectiveness of the program.

DISCUSSION

While the project was both interesting and challenging, a great deal of time was required–at least 400 hours. Working with a group of six involved many calendars, drafts, and deadlines. Although the advertisements for authoring packages would have one believe that CAI programs can be created quickly and easily, this is not realistic. Two separate reviews of Authorware products echo this sentiment. Tessler, writing about *Course of Action,* states:

> The documentation is among the best I've seen for any type of software, guiding you through all the steps with plenty of examples. Still, creating effective instructional software isn't an easy process–expect many hours of hard work for every hour of courseware.[6]

Poage agrees with this assessment in a review of *Authorware Professional:*

> The authors state ease-of-use as a major goal, and I feel they have accomplished this without sacrificing quality. However, this is not a program for beginning computer users. Creating sophisticated CAI is not a simple task . . . it remains a very complex application.[7]

Is it practical to produce CAI in-house for use in library user education? The answer to this question is, of course, not clear-cut. Many hours of staff time were required to produce a product that runs for approximately 45 minutes. Recent library literature reaffirms the value of teaching and learning about MeSH. Marshall found that, among end-user searchers, "Frequency of MeSH use is associated with more positive perceptions of online searching. . . . These results confirm the importance of continuing to teach the use of MeSH."[8] Similarly, Kirby and Miller found that effective use of MeSH contributed significantly to the success of end-user searches.[9] The challenge is to convince users that it is worthwhile for them to spend the time necessary to learn MeSH, even at a basic level. *Watch Your Language* teaches the basics of MeSH in 45 minutes. Ideally, an advanced program should be available to teach *Annotated MeSH*.

This brings up a further question: Is CAI a good format for teaching MeSH to library users? In order to make the most effective use of the interactive aspect of CAI, it would be necessary to break MeSH down into a series of very specific concepts with a set of questions for each concept. There are so many important concepts in MeSH that the resulting program would be very long. Since many hours of intense work are required to produce one hour of instruction, it would be a big commitment to produce such a product. The real stumbling block, however, is convincing library users to take advantage of such a product.

CONCLUSION

In conclusion, a number of statements can be made regarding MeSH, *Watch Your Language,* and CAI. Design and production of this program demonstrated in a real way that MeSH is an extremely complex tool which is not possible to learn in a few minutes. MeSH may be less important in the future if search systems become so sophisticated that a searcher can effectively retrieve information using natural language. For the present, librarians continue to look for novel ways to teach MeSH.

Watch Your Language is an innovative way to teach MeSH, using CAI technology to create an engaging program. The staff at SML looks forward to incorporating the product into user education activities and to sharing it with both end users and other librarians. The next decision to be made concerns whether to use the skills gained during this project to work on a new CAI program or whether to enhance the existing program by adding an interactive question section to each appropriate module. It might then be more feasible to use the program module by module, as needed, rather than as a complete introduction to MeSH. A patron who is confused about cross-references, for example, could be directed to the appropriate module and questions at the point of need.

Producing a CAI program is a sophisticated activity that involves an enormous amount of time. Given the diversity of skills and the amount of time needed, the team approach appears to be an effective way to produce a complete program. Successful creation of CAI requires not only a thorough knowledge of the topic but also requires an entirely new way of thinking about the known material. Although not to be undertaken lightly, producing CAI programs in-house can be a challenging and rewarding experience for library staff.

APPENDIX

READINGS IN COMPUTER-ASSISTED INSTRUCTION

1. Alessi, Stephen M., and Trollip, Stanley R. *Computer-Based Instruction: Methods and Development.* Englewood Cliffs, NJ: Prentice-Hall, 1985.

2. *Apple Guide to Courseware Authoring.* Cupertino, CA: Apple Computer, 1988.

3. Billings, Diane M. *Computer Assisted Instruction for Health Professionals: A Guide to Designing and Using CAI Courseware.* Norwalk, CT: Appleton-Century-Crofts, 1986.

4. Heines, Jesse M. *Screen Design Strategies for Computer-Aided Instruction.* Bedford, MA: Digital Press, 1984.

5. Jonassen, David H. *Instructional Designs for Microcomputer Courseware.* Hillsdale, NJ: Lawrence Erlbaum Associates, 1988,

6. _____ . *The Technology of Text: Principles for Structuring, Designing, and Displaying Text.* Englewood Cliffs, NJ: Educational Technology Publications, 1982.

7. Kearsley, Greg. *Artificial Intelligence and Instruction.* Reading, MA: Addison, Wesley, 1987.

8. _____ . *Authoring: A Guide to the Design of Instructional Software.* Reading, MA: Addison-Wesley, 1986.

9. _____ . *Online Help Systems: Design and Implementation.* Norwood, NJ: Ablex, 1988.

10. Shneiderman, Ben. *Designing the User Interface: Strategies for Effective Human-Computer Interaction.* Reading, MA: Addison-Wesley, 1987.

11. Walker, Decker F., and Hess, Robert D. *Instructional Software: Principles and Perspectives for Design and Use.* Belmont, CA: Wadsworth, 1984.

PREVIOUS CAI PROGRAMS FEATURING MeSH

1. *MEDLEARN.* Bethesda, MD: National Library of Medicine, circa 1985.

2. *Searching the Biomedical Literature: A Comprehensive Computer-Assisted Instructional Program.* Cincinnati, OH: University of Cincinnati Medical Center, Medical Center Information and Communications, 1985.

3. *Tutorial Number 2: MEDLINE.* Scotia, NY: BRS Colleague, May 1985.

REFERENCES

1. Joint Task Force of the Association of Academic Health Sciences Library Directors and the Medical Library Association. *Challenge to Action: Planning and Evaluation Guidelines for Academic Health Sciences Libraries.* Chicago: Medical Library Association, 1987.

2. Piemme, Thomas E. "Computer-Assisted Learning and Evaluation in Medicine." *Journal of the American Medical Association* 260 (July 15, 1988):367-372.

3. The Health Sciences Libraries Consortium is a cooperative of Pennsylvania and Delaware medical school and health sciences research libraries. Based in Philadelphia, the Consortium is funded in part by a major grant from the Pew Charitable Trusts.

4. *Course of Action™.* Minneapolis: Authorware, Inc., 1988.

5. *Apple Guide to Courseware Authoring.* Cupertino CA: Apple Computer, 1988.

6. Tessler, Franklin. "Courseware to Go: *Course of Action* 1.0, The Best *Course of Action* 1.0." *Macworld* 5 (Sept. 1988):221-222.

7. Poage, Julie A. *"Course of Action."* *Computing Teacher* 16 (February 1, 1989):40-42.

8. Marshall, Joanne G. "End-User Training: Does It Make a Difference?" *Medical Reference Services Quarterly* 8 (Fall 1989):15-25.

9. Kirby, Martha Z., and Miller, Naomi. "MEDLINE Searching on Colleague: Reasons for Failure or Success of Untrained End Users." *Medical Reference Services Quarterly* 5 (Fall 1986):17-34.

Chapter 27

A Sam Starr Mystery:
Building a Computerized Tour
for the Library

Dan Sienkiewicz
Melinda Buckwalter
helen-ann brown

Cornell Medical Library, like many other academic health science center libraries, is traditionally busy in the fall conducting orientation tours. What could be done to complement these overview walking tours of the Library? What kind of library orientation could be offered year-round? What tool could be made available to help answer a quick question about the location of a library office or an item in the collection, or to review Cornell Medical Library policies, programs, and services?

"A Sam Starr Mystery–The Quest for Knowledge" is a computer tour that was created to meet this need. During the fall orientation tour, Sam Starr would be demonstrated, and then throughout the year library staff could direct library patrons to the computer on which Sam Starr was mounted. Sam Starr would also be accessible to users outside the Library via the New York Hospital-Cornell Medical Center (NYH-CMC) network.

This chapter was first published in *Medical Reference Services Quarterly*, Vol. 13(4), Winter 1994.

Helen-ann brown, Head of Library Relations, coordinated this project. With Dan Sienkiewicz from Library Computer Services and Melinda Buckwalter of the Media Desk staff, she formed the core Sam Starr team. The core team began to meet weekly on Friday afternoons. They chose to create the tour in the Macintosh program HyperCard for several reasons: Cornell Medical Library is predominantly a Macintosh world; HyperCard has the ability to combine hypertext and graphics, including animation; it is easy to use; and it is modestly priced. The team looked at other HyperCard programs that gave a library tour or introduced a product or service. They found entertaining programs to be the most successful in holding people's interest. Therefore, they decided to make their tour entertaining as well as informative.

One Friday afternoon at the end of a hectic week, the theme for the tour was born–a detective as a tour guide to lead the search for information. Brown solicited the library staff for drawings of this character. She envisioned the detective to be dashing, in a trench coat with his hat pulled low. Sienkiewicz created such a character. At first he looked more like Hercule Poirot than Bogart; however, Sienkiewicz slimmed him down, and added height and mysterious shades. Other entries came from Buckwalter who created a Cybil Shepherd-like woman and a dog, both capped and caped like Sherlock Holmes. The characters' names, Sam Starr, C. Victoria, and Woody, originated as plays on the official name of the Library–The Samuel J. Wood Library/C. V. Starr Biomedical Information Center (see Figure 27.1).

The team now turned their attention to the tour's structure. They wanted to cover general information such as library hours, loan periods, and locations of public phones. They also wanted a user to be able to conduct his or her own tour of the library by clicking on computer screen maps. The last objective was to introduce library users to Cornell Medical Library's programs and services. To meet these objectives, the team decided the tour should have three main sections or stacks: Quick Tour, General Information, and Library Services. They also planned to include a help and credits section.

Once the general theme and the structure of the tour had been decided upon, the team divided up responsibilities. Sienkiewicz would learn more about HyperCard, design the basic card layout, and develop the Quick Tour section. Buckwalter would design the animations. Brown would gather the text for the General Information and Library Services sections.

DESIGN AND TECHNICAL DEVELOPMENT

Sienkiewicz had some prior knowledge of HyperCard, so he was not starting completely from scratch. He found that the most useful way to learn was by taking apart other people's stacks and seeing how they had put them together. He used a few books to augment his knowledge (see suggested reading list), especially *HyperCard 2 in a Hurry.* He found the HyperCard Listserv on the Internet to be immensely helpful. If he ran into technical problems he posted his problem to the list and a helpful suggestion or answer would be posted within hours.

In designing the card layout, Sienkiewicz used many concepts from hypertext and human-computer interface design books. The idea was to have the graphic elements of the interface, like the buttons, be simple with enough information so that their function would be clear to the user. He wanted the interface, the way the user interacts with the program, to be unobtrusive so that the text areas, graphics, or animation could come forward and express the main ideas and action of the tour. The interface would then serve as a frame for the graphics and text and ideally become more transparent as the user went through the tour.

Sienkiewicz decided that a button panel similar to the control panel of a VCR would be best. Since most people are right-handed, Sienkiewicz put the button panel on the right vertical side of the screen. This offered the least amount of mouse movement in accessing the buttons and left more active area for the text and graphics.

In building the interface, it was important to take into account the different levels of users' knowledge of HyperCard. The most effective interface would be geared toward the majority of users while taking into consideration differences and variety within that group. The team found they constantly needed to put themselves in the mind of the user. This helped them avoid making assumptions that could confuse the users.

In developing the Quick Tour section, Sienkiewicz used the tour

FIGURE 27.1. Main Screen Introducing Sam, C. Victoria, and Woody

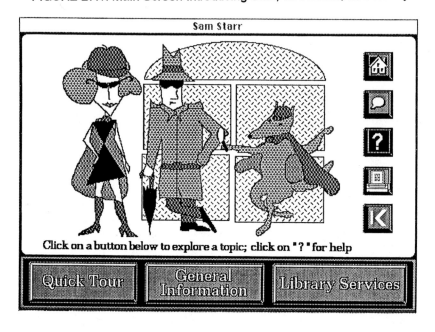

of the library at the Washington University Health Sciences Center as a model. The Cornell Medical Library floor plans were already computerized. Several more detailed floor plans were drawn to expand on areas of specific interest.

ANIMATION

Buckwalter's first decision in developing the animations was in which program to work. Sienkiewicz had researched various animation programs that could interface with HyperCard and recommended the inexpensive, easy-to-use Animation Works. Buckwalter agreed and completed the tutorial before experimenting. She soon realized the drawing capabilities of Animation Works were limited. Instead she drew in Adobe Illustrator and then imported the drawings into Animation Works to create the animation. Adobe Illustrator is an object-oriented graphics program that works on an anchor point concept. This made portions of objects easy to copy and transform–an obvious advantage when animating.

Buckwalter's first animation of C. Victoria kneeling taught her a lot. The kneeling animation required distortion of the legs as they bent and an angling of the torso. When she finished, the animation was about ten frames, but it was not as smooth as she would have liked. For a beginner it was just too hard and time-consuming to redraw and make the animation look smooth.

Buckwalter learned to simplify fast. The trick was to imagine movements that would require copying and displacement of the object rather than a distortion. An example of this simple type of animation is a dog running, made of two pictures. One picture is of the dog with his legs out and the second with his legs gathered under him. Alternating the two pictures and displacing it across a background gives the dog the illusion of movement (see Figure 27.2). Other examples of simple animation are a car driving across the screen, eyes moving back and forth, and a scarf flapping in the wind. These were quick to make and added interest to the screens without over-complicating them.

Buckwalter developed eight mini-movies with moving players and background scenery. When the team began to incorporate these animations into the HyperCard stack, they ran into major problems. First, the load time for the animations was too long. The stack was mainly for information gathering; they did not want any lag time in its access. Second, the animations were too self-contained as they had been developed. The team wanted them to be more integrated into the tour itself, not as a separate feature.

To correct the first problem Buckwalter decided not to use the Animation Works program and go with the simple flip book animation approach. HyperCard lends itself to this idea since it is, after all, just a virtual stack of cards. Sienkiewicz showed Buckwalter how to write a script in HyperCard that made it flip through a specified number of cards. The computer could also be scripted to play a sound. There was now no load time, since all the animating was done by HyperCard itself. Since Buckwalter had all the drawings, she just had to copy them onto cards in HyperCard. Even though she ended up not using Animation Works, Buckwalter felt it had been a great practice and development tool. The manual had

FIGURE 27.2. A Simple Animation Sequence

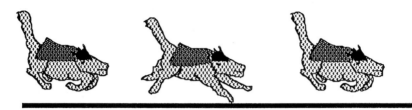

lots of tips about animating. Animation Works also simplifies the task of animating, which is great for beginners.

The second separate feature problem was a conceptual one. Buckwalter realized she needed to deconstruct her movies and integrate individual players into the stack. Instead of having the movie play as a separate item at the beginning of a section, the new version had the actors appearing alongside the text itself. The animation now had the effect the team intended, to add interest to the stack without interfering with the main goal–information retrieval.

GATHERING THE TEXT

Brown was responsible for gathering the text. Text for the General Information Section was taken from an information card developed by Circulation to distribute to new users. Brown filled in additional information when needed. The team had already decided the first card for each program area would include an overview statement, list of staff names, and phone numbers. Brown met with the head of each program area and asked what facts each wanted to include in his or her stack for the Library Services Section. Some departments wrote their own copy, while others gave Brown ideas from which she wrote the text.

PUTTING THE TOUR TOGETHER

One of the most time-consuming parts of the project was organizing the text that Brown gathered into stacks. How should the cards flow? How should information be cross-referenced? Sienkie-wicz insisted on consistency in the design of the cards and of the user interface. This consistency would help the user with rudimentary knowledge of HyperCard to be able to navigate successfully through the stacks.

Buckwalter took on this problem and started with her own department, since she knew its structure best. She made a flowchart of her department, moving from the general to the specific. Sometimes one topic would generate multiple topics. Here she would place a button card in the HyperCard stack, with a button for each of the topics. Some departments proved to be linear by nature, one card moving naturally to the next. These sections could be moved through with a *next* button that stepped through the stack in order. Other departments' flowcharts were full of jumping points–button cards with multiple topic options as destinations. Clearly the team needed to allow for both type of activities.

Cross-referencing also created a need for buttons. The team wanted to allow the user to hop back and forth between the three major sections. This created a thorny logic problem. They went to other HyperCard stacks to see how others handled the combination of movements they wanted to allow: linear travel, hierarchical (jumping) travel, and cross-referencing. They did not find one stack that solved all their problems so they borrowed from each and invented when needed. It would have saved them considerable time if they had foreseen these problems. As it was, about halfway through the project they realized that they needed a retrace button, a button that would allow returning after a jump. This meant redesigning the button panel that appeared on every card.

It was also very important for each button to be consistent in its function; there should be no surprises for the user. Often this meant repetition of function–buttons going to the same card at certain points in the tour. Another question that arose was whether a button should be left out entirely or just disabled if it had no function in a particular context. The team's answer was to create dimmed buttons that kept the visual consistency of the interface. Eventually the team developed a consistent interface that allowed for all the types of movement they had established (see Figure 27.3).

FIGURE 27.3. Sample Card Showing Interface

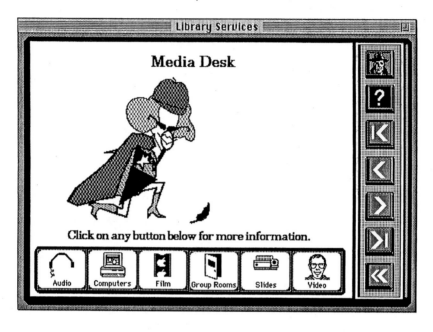

RECOMMENDATIONS

Computer expertise, drawing talent, and layout and conceptual design skills are necessary to build a tour. A team allows for divided responsibility and exchange of ideas. This team found HyperCard to be a versatile vehicle for designing a tour and keeping the information up-to-date.

The team found the creation of the interface to be the most time-consuming and difficult aspect of the tour. Flowcharts for specific areas proved helpful. Time could have been saved by making a flowchart for the entire tour. A general flowchart could have predicted what movements would be needed and would have helped to develop a consistent approach. Several redesigns could have been avoided.

The team was pleased with the finished product and has received positive feedback from staff members, library colleagues, and library patrons. Good luck to future HyperCard tour builders!

SUGGESTED READING LIST

Animation

1. *Animation Works User Guide.* Mississagua, Ontario, Canada: Gold Disk, 1990.
2. Laybourne, Kit. *The Animation Book.* New York: Crown, 1979.

Computers and Multimedia

1. Laurel, Brenda. *Computers as Theater.* Redding, MA: Addison-Wesley, 1993.
2. Laurel, Brenda, editor. *Art of Human-Computer Interface Design.* Redding, MA: Addison-Wesley, 1990.

HyperCard

1. Beekman, George. *HyperCard 2 in a Hurry.* Belmont, CA: Wadsworth, 1992.
2. Coulouris, George, Thimbleby, Harold. *Hyperprogramming.* Redding, MA: Addison-Wesley, 1993.
3. Goodman, Danny. *The Complete HyperCard Handbook.* 2nd ed. New York: Bantam Books, 1988.

Internet Resources

1. To subscribe to the HyperCard Listserv send a message to LISTSERV@MSU.BITNET with a blank subject line and the text of the message containing: SUBSCRIBE HYPERCRD FirstName LastName.
2. UseNet Mailing List: comp.sys.mac.hypercard.

Index

Academic health sciences libraries
surveys, 159-165,167-175
Adobe Illustrator, 284-285
Allegri, Francesca, 35-41
American Association of Medical
Colleges, 229
American College of Physicians,
229
American Library Association, 159-
160
Antoniewicz, Carol M., 209-219
ASKSAM, 211-216,218
Association of Academic Health
Sciences Library Directors,
173,267
Association of College and Research
Libraries *Guidelines,* 160,164
Asu, Glynis Vandoorne, 209-219
Audiovisual aids. *See* Videotapes

BI-L, 58
Bibliographic instruction
history of, 8
in hospital library, 87-92
BIOSIS, 123
BOOKENDS, 211
Boolean logic, 66,89,101-102,
129,169,171-173,184-185,
249,251
brown, helen-ann, 281-289
BRS, 110-112,177
BRS Colleague, 80,118,137,177,
224,226,250
BRS SearchMate, 177
Bryant, Joyce, 267-280
Buckwalter, Melinda, 281-289
Burnham, Judy F., 237-254

Cahan, Mitchell Aaron, 221-227
Calabretta, Nancy, 267-280
Canadian Health Libraries
Association, 124
Canadian Institute for Scientific
and Technical Information,
124,128
Canadian Medical Association,
124,127
CD Plus MEDLINE, 92,95-107,275
author searching, 103-104
browsing, 102-103
combining sets, 101-102
demonstration, 80,89
instruction, 80,90-91,95-107
journal title searching, 104-106
subject searching, 97-100
Text Word searching, 100-101
CD Plus Plusnet, 80,83-84
CD-ROM, 91,123,126,135,147,204
CD-ROM MEDLINE, 109-112.
See also CD Plus MEDLINE;
Compact Cambridge MEDLINE
instruction, 167-175,202-203;
See also End-user searching
surveys, 167-175
Chiang, Dudee, 109-115
CINAHL, 80,88,242-243,245-246,
250-251,272
Clancy, Stephen, 61-77
Clinical consulting. *See* Consultation
services
Clinical medical librarian program,
28,33
Collins, Barbara, 229-236
Compact Cambridge MEDLINE,
109,137-138

291

Educational programs, program
goals *(continued)*
surveys, 159-165
Educational services.
See Educational programs
Electronic bulletin boards, 205-206
EMBASE, 123
End-user searching, 117-122,123-
133,135-149
and mediated searches, 137-141,
143,183,185
evaluation of instruction, 177-186
implementation, 126-128
instruction, 95-107,117-122,123-
133,144-146,167-175,178-
180; See also instruction
subheading under CD-ROM
MEDLINE, CD Plus MED-
LINE, Grateful MED, MED-
LINE, USCInfo MEDLINE
management of services, 146-148
role of librarian, 135-149
surveys, 123-133,167-175
training methods, 124-128,169-
172
transactional logs, 180-186
End users
attitudes, 130-132
success rates, 181-186
surveys, 123-133
use of MeSH, 128-131,178,
182-186

Feldman, Jonquil D., 79-85

General Professional Education
for Physicians (GPEP)
Report, 61,247
George Washington University
Medical Center, Himmelfarb
Health Sciences Library,
230-236
Glick, Jacqueline, 209-219

Grateful MED, 80,88,109,111,132,
185,226
instruction, 90-91,163-164,202,
224,226,242,244,245-246,
248,250
Gresehover, Beverly A., 87-92

HEALTH, 80
Health Sciences Libraries
Consortium (HSLC),
268-269
Hopkins Current Contents, 226
Hospital libraries, 87-92
Housecalls, 79-85. See also
Information management
education program
development, 80-82
Housestaff
orientations, 88-89
research techniques, 89-90
Hypercard, 282-288,289
Hypertext, 269,272-273,277,282-289

Index Medicus, 110,242,245-246,
248-251,259,275
Information fair, 232-234
Information literacy
defined, 237. See also Computer
literacy
Information management education,
202-204,222,237-254.
See also Personal file
management software
costs of, 28,33
course content, 28-30,202-204,
242-251
course-integrated instruction,
33,238-239
history of, 8-9
instructional objectives, 242-251
program development, 80-82,
240-242
review of, 62-64
role of librarian, 189-195,209-219